Sociology of Health

Sociology of Health

Mohammad Akram

RAWAT PUBLICATIONS

Jaipur • New Delhi • Bangalore • Hyderabad • Guwahati • Kolkata

ISBN 978-81-316-0558-5

Reprinted, 2017

Published by
Prem Rawat for **Rawat Publications**
Satyam Apts, Sector 3, Jawahar Nagar, Jaipur 302 004 (India)
Phone: 0141 265 1748 / 7006 Fax: 0141 265 1748
E-mail: info@rawatbooks.com
Website: www.rawatbooks.com

New Delhi Office
4858/24, Ansari Road, Daryaganj, New Delhi 110 002
Phone: 011 2326 3290

Also at *Bangalore, Guwahati* and *Kolkata*

Typeset by Rawat Computers, Jaipur
Printed at Chaman Enterprises, New Delhi

Contents

Preface

A global academic framework is necessary for understanding sociology and especially sociologically. This holds true not only for the classical sociology which developed in Europe and America by the end of nineteenth and early twentieth century, but also for the various sub-disciplines of sociology developed or developing in various other parts of the world. Sociology of health (or medical sociology in different contexts) drew the attention of researchers and policy makers as an important sub-discipline of sociology in the West and the rest of the world by the early decades of the second half of the twentieth century. The Alma Ata Declaration of 1978 made 'health for all' a universal goal and brought 'health' at the core of the development agenda in the welfare economies. Subsequently, health became an integral component of human development. The 'social determinants of health' approach challenged the hegemony of the 'biomedical determinism' in explaining illness and disease and the social sciences responded to provide not only supplementary but also alternative explanations for prevailing poor health conditions in various parts of the world. Sociology of health finds its ground in India under these circumstances.

At a different level, my participation in the World Congress of Sociology, 2010, held at Gotenborg, Sweden, and interactions in Research Committee 15 (Sociology of Health) exposed me to the profound popularity of sociology of health and medical sociology as sub-discipline of sociology in various universities and research institutes at global level. Way back in India, my experience as Convener of Research Committee 12 (Health, Population, and Society) of Indian Sociological Society made me realize that 'sociology of health, disease, and health care' is attracting the students and researchers at pan-India level. Most of the universities are promoting research and courses on various issues that broadly come under sociology of health. The interventions made by the United Nations, World Health Organization (WHO), and other global agencies in promoting health care also play significant role in that. The concept of health and its possible dimensions are gradually being redefined. Right to health and health care is the new aspiration of people. Sociology of health as a sub-discipline of sociology is reflecting this shift of paradigm in health and health care very well.

The exposure of people in India to systematically introduced processes, such as globalization, liberalization, and privatization, within the broader framework of 'structural adjustment programmes' in the last decade of the past century created new opportunities and challenges. The information revolution exposed people not only to the advancement made in social and human developments in the rest of world, but it also made people realize the poor achievements in our own country under these parameters. The rise of the 'third sector' (broadly including non-governmental organizations, civil society groups, community organizations, etc.) in the age of 'democratic decentralization' and 'right to information' heralds the beginning of a new interest in public policy and development planning. Governance is no longer an issue confined to political elites or bureaucratic managers; common people have also started taking interest in it and the demand of transparency is the new aspiration. Sociology of health is increasingly reflecting this new endeavour in academic and public spheres.

My continuous interaction with students and research scholars at various levels has exposed me to another felt problem of sociology students in India—the lack of comprehensive texts on 'sociology of health in India'. Students generally look for standard texts that can provide information on the theoretical perspectives as well as the empirical realities in Indian context. We have very standard textbooks available from authors such as William C. Cockerham; Sarah Nettleton; David Mechanic; Sol Levine; M. Stacey (with H. Homans); Richard K. Thomas; Bryan S. Turner; Kelvin White; Chris Yuill; Mary Larkin; S. Kelman; Diana Kendall; U. Gerhardt; R. Dingwall; Peter Conrad; K. Park; Rodney M. Coe; J.F. McKenzie, R.R. Pinger and J.E. Kotecki; Jonathan Gabe, Mike Bury, and Mary Elson; E. Hansen and G. Easthop; C. Miller, B. Waning, J. Bread and A. Knapp, and many more. We do have good published research works in India by authors such as Aneeta Minocha, D. Banerji, Rama V. Baru, Imrana Qadeer, Madhu Nagla, K.R. Nayar, Reema Bhatia, T.N. Madan, M. Akram, Indranil Mukopadhyay, Tulsi Patel, V. Sujatha, R. Venkataratnam, S.R. Mehta, and many more. However, there is an absolute lack of text that can fulfil the needs of a student or a beginner by providing a broad theoretical and conceptual framework with its focus on Indian health scenario. This book is intended to fill this gap.

This book takes a comprehensive approach on health: it goes beyond the boundaries and limitations of medical sociology, social medicine or community health. Medical sociology, in its approach, is narrowly centred on or around the medical institutions in general. Health in India is much more than medical intervention. India is characterized by medical pluralism: it includes the conventional or traditional medicine, folk medicine, modern medical interventions and much more. Disease in India has much wider implications than what they imply in modern western countries. Communicable disease is still responsible for millions of pre-mature mortalities. Malnutrition and lack of safe drinking water are compounding the problem many times more. Environmental degradation, sanitation, and poor living conditions create huge handicaps. There is a wide variation in morbidity, mortality, and health care patterns in India. The health indicators suggest wide prevalence of health inequality within and between the states. This book covers all such issues in a thorough manner.

There are several reports and documents submitted by various expert committees constituted by the Government of India responding to various needs and requirements. Most of such reports remain beyond the purview or reach of the students. This book has also referred to a good number of such reports and presented the relevant contents in a systematic way under various headings and sub-headings, as and when required. Such reports are not just reflection of the views of the experts of the panels, but they also ultimately decide the direction of public policy and health planning processes. The Bhore Committee Report in pre-independent India largely decided the direction of health care in the country. Although the report was never implemented in totality, but still it is a vision document for health planning in India. The health structure developed in the last six decades does reflect the views of many such reports. One recent report submitted for attaining the goals of 'universal health coverage' will have its impact for decades.

Privatization of health is an important policy shift in India. The government's share in the health care sector is only about 20 per cent. The rest is shared by the private sector. The last decade of the past century witnessed a huge shift towards privatization of health care. The burden of health care is increasing fast. Most of the cost of treatment is met by 'out-of-pocket' expenditures. This has created huge inequalities in health outcomes. The impact of health inequality is multidimensional and long-lasting. Most of the time the government's initiatives cause more inequalities than minimizing them. The reforms suggested through National Rural Health Mission, Rashtriya Suraksha Bima Yojana, etc., in the aftermath of Millennium Development Goals, have limited outcomes.

This book is an effort to address most of these issues. The 16 chapters have tried to address the prevailing diversities of the views and perspectives in sociology of health by including and frequently quoting many of the popular authors. The purpose is to make the beginners aware of the existing writings and present the things in simplest words. Complete references are given for each chapter. Select bibliography given at the end serves two purposes: introducing the students with the esteemed works of the authors and acknowledging the support that has been taken from them in preparing this manuscript. The author has also quoted from his own published works frequently giving proper references and making due acknowledgements. Any omission in providing proper references anywhere in this book is purely accidental and duly apologized by the author.

I would like to share the credit of this work with all the authors, co-authors and publishers, whose views and ideas have been included in various chapters of this book. I am indebted to all of them. I would like to acknowledge the support of various experts, panelists and co-panelists in various conferences at national and international level for helping me to shape my own views on various issues during the presentation of various research papers. I am equally thankful to the critics who helped me to improve my own works. My students and research scholars deserve special appreciation for mentally preparing me to take this endeavour. Zulufkar Ahmad Khanday needs special thanks for undertaking much of the pain related to this work. Without his hard work, it was never possible to complete the work. The love and affection of my parents, Mohammad Naimuddin and Noor Dana Khatoon, is always a source of strength for me. And last, but not the least, I am indebted to my wife Firdousi, son Arshad, and daughter Alveena for their full support in every possible way. I am extremely thankful to Rawat Publications for undertaking the publication of this book.

I look forward for your views and comments. I am sure your comments will enrich the quality of the book in its next edition.

Chapter One

Sociology of Health

Definition, Emergence, and Phases

During the early years of emergence of sociology as a discipline, the founding fathers studied institutions such as family, religion, economic system, political system, and other social institutions. Till the early twentieth century, sociology hardly included the health care institution as an area of study. According to Thomas, 'health care was neglected because it had yet to emerge as a full-blown social institution. For this reason, medical sociology as an accepted field did not emerge until after Second World War nor did it achieve any significant development until the 1960s. Consequently, medical sociology matured in an intellectual climate far different from nineteenth and early twentieth-century environment that spawned early social thought' (2002: 07).

'Sociology offers a variety of means to understand the incidence and experience of illness and health within societies as well as the social organization of the delivery of health care and differential access to health care resources. The specific application of sociology to the field of health, illness and health care has been termed as medical sociology' (Raphael, Bryant, and Rioux, 2006: 35). In the words of David Mechanic, 'medical sociology is an interdisciplinary field that benefits richly not only from the work of sociologists and social psychologists but also from that of researchers in medicine and public health, epidemiologists, health economists and physicians involved in researching their own practices' (1978: vii). According to De Maio (2010), medical sociology is interested in the causes of diseases, its distribution, and ways of controlling its spread in population. Cockerham states that 'medical sociology is the study of the social causes and consequences of health and illness' (2007: 32). Thus, medical sociology cuts across many traditional areas of sociological inquiry and sociologists who work in this field have differing interests and motivations.

Tracing the development of medical sociology, Scambler (1987) opines that medical sociology is normally regarded as post-Second World War phenomenon, and as originating in the United States. But in Europe, and especially in France, Germany, and Britain, social aspects of health and disease had been studied within disciplines such as social medicine, public health and anthropology since the late eighteenth century. Scambler says that modern medical sociology in Britain and most other European countries bears the stamp of its antecedent or 'premodern' phase. However, the genesis of medical sociology was very different in the United States. It began to grow shortly after the Second World War (for further discussion, see Akram, 2012).

Robert Straus (1957) best summarizes the direction taken by medical sociology in its early development. Straus suggests that medical sociology is divided into two separate but closely interrelated areas: sociology *of* medicine and sociology *in* medicine. Cockerham and Ritchey (1997) in 'Dictionary of Medical Sociology' state that 'sociology of medicine deals with such factors as the organization, role relationships, norms, values, and beliefs of medical practice as a form of human behaviour (Straus, 1957). The emphasis is on the social processes that occur in the medical setting and how these contribute to our understanding of medical sociology in particular and to our understanding of social life in general. The sociology of medicine shares the same goals as all other areas of sociology and may consequently be characterized as research and analysis of the medical environment from a sociological perspective. Thus, the sociology of medicine can be characterized as primarily motivated by the solution of sociological problems rather than medical problems. Although some sociologists of medicine are employed in health institutions, the majority work as professors in the sociology departments of universities and colleges' (Cockerham and Ritchey, 1997: 122–123).

According to Turner, 'sociology of medicine is seen as less oriented to the professional interests of medicine and treats the concepts of health and illness as problematic and constructed. Medicine itself is studied as an institution and practice, and there is concern with the issue of power relations between doctors and patients. The larger term, the sociology of health and illness, defines the concept positively and includes not only the profession of medicine, but also the whole range of caring occupations and activities, and not only the identification, treatment, and experience of illness, but also health-related lifestyles and health as general well-being' (2006: 261).

According to Cockerham and Ritchey (1997) sociologist *in* medicine is a sociologist who collaborates directly with physicians and other health personnel in studying the social factors that are relevant to a particular health problem. The work of the sociologist in medicine is intended to be directly applicable to patient care and other practical uses in the area of health. Thus, sociology in medicine is characterized as applied research and analysis primarily motivated by a medical problem rather than a sociological problem. Some of the tasks of the sociologist in medicine are to analyse the causes of health disorders; the differences in social attitudes as they relate to health; and the ways in which the incidence and prevalence of a specific health disorder are related to social variables such as age, sex, socio-economic status, racial/ethnic group identity, education, and occupation.

Raphael, Bryant, and Rioux (2006) also join the debate and explain that sociologists *in* medicine usually work in medical schools, nursing schools, public health schools, teaching hospitals, public health agencies, and other health organizations. They may also work for a governmental agency such as the US Department of Health and Human Services or the Centres for Disease Control and Prevention in the capacity of biostatisticians, health planners, administrators, and other positions. According to Raphael, Bryant, and Rioux, 'this reflects a movement away from a medically defined approach to one that is more theoretically oriented, deriving its inspiration—much like the rest of sociology—from the founding traditions of Durkheim, Weber, and Marx and more recently from feminist, anti-racism, and postmodernist scholars. While the distinction between sociology *in* and *of* is important to make, it is difficult to tease apart these orientations in practice because many medical sociologists are engaged both in advancing sociology through insights garnered from health and health care and in using their knowledge to create practical change' (2006: 36).

'The use of the term 'medical sociology' has been noted as early as 1894 in an article by Charles McIntire on the importance of social factors in health' (Thomas, 2002: 8). 'As it was first developed in the Anglophone world, medical sociology (as the sub-discipline was first named and the term which is still preferred in the United States) or the sociology of health and illness (the term preferred in Britain and Australia) was primarily concerned with systematic empiricism using the measurement of objective variables deemed quantifiable'(italics added) (Lupton, 2003: 6). Thomas further says, 'the recognition of the complex relationships between social factors and the level of health and disease characteristic of various groups, as was noticed by increasing number of sociologists, has made an important substantive development within the general field of sociology: the growth of 'sociology of health and illness' as a separate branch of sociology. Just as sociology is concerned with the social causes and consequences of human behaviour, similarly the 'sociology of health and illness' is concerned with the social causes and consequences of health and illness' (Thomas, 2002: 8). Gradually, according to Turner, ''sociology of health and illness' is now the preferred term, suggesting a wider canvas than the purely 'medical', though medical sociology is still often used for convenience' (Turner, 2006: 261).

Sociology of health includes a wide territory of issues: how some conditions came to be called diseases; the experience of being sick or ill; the organization of the medical profession; the ways in which health policies are developed; and the working of hospitals. In all these areas, sociological studies of health and disease provide microcosms of the working of the wider society. Thus, sociologists are interested in health and disease not as health practitioners, but as students of society. The sociology of health brings sociological perspectives, theories, and methods to the study of health and health care. Following are reasons to study the sociology of health: (1) Sociologists are not trying to tell health practitioners how to do their job, though some of their findings can tell us interesting things about how medicine and nursing are practiced. (2) The focus is not on the individual as such but on the group of which individual is the member. Thus, the sociologists' perspective is not on the individual as such but on the group to which they belong. For a sociologist what people get sick of, how they are treated, and why they die of is a product not of their personality or primarily of their biology, but of their position in a set of power relationships that are formed out of access to these goods which guarantee the quality of life. (3) To see the ways in which we label and treat illnesses as a form of social control (White, 2009: 40–41).

According to Larkin (2011), sociology of health and illness has now achieved professional and academic recognition. As a result of its further development and sociological underpinnings, it is concerned with all aspects of contemporary life that impose on well-being throughout the life course. Examples of the wide range of issues that the sociology of health and illness currently addresses are as follows:

1. Patterns of health and illness in relation to the wider social structure.
2. Lay perceptions of health and illness.
3. The experience of health and illness.
4. How certain conditions come to be viewed as illnesses or diseases?
5. Globalization and health.
6. The social organization of formal and informal health care.
7. The analysis of medical knowledge and professional power.
8. Lay-professional interactions in health care.
9. The social and cultural aspects of the body.

In exploring these issues, the sociology of health and illness adopts a diverse approach and it embraces other disciplines, such as epidemiology, public health, social policy, and psychology. It also employs many well-established sociological perspectives in its explanations. Clarke (1981) has given different perspectives to study contents of sociology of health. He makes a distinction between positivists (whose aim is to discover causal laws), activists (whose aim is to diagnose societies' ills and propose solutions), and naturalists (whose aim is empathetically to interpret the meaning of situations). Gerhardt (1989) classifies the contents of sociology of health and illness within four theoretical paradigms: structural functionalism, symbolic interactionism, phenomenology, and conflict theory. Turner (2006) suggests the levels of analysis approach for understanding health and illness sociologically. He suggests study of health and illness in society at three levels: the 'individual level', which examines perceptions of health and illness; the 'social level', which examines the social creation of disease categories and health care organizations; and the 'societal level', which examines the health care systems within their political context. Further, according to Kevin White (2002), different sociological perspectives on society give rise to different accounts of the role of medical knowledge, and of the social causes of disease. White has examined some of the popular perspectives of sociology of health separately.

The Marxist approach talks more about disease than health, emphasizing the causal role of economics in the production and distribution of disease. It also emphasizes the role that medical knowledge plays in sustaining the class structure. Parsonian sociology, having functional approach, emphasizes the role of medicine in maintaining social harmony by pointing to the non-market basis of professional groups. Parsons' work not only contradicts Marxism—by highlighting the importance of the non-economic sphere of society—but also adds to it in providing a description of the sick role as a social role that is shaped by the social strains of modern society. Foucault's work (1973), in particular, 'The Birth of Clinic', is a sustained attempt to analyse medical knowledge as a product of specific historical period. His central argument is that modern medicine is a manifestation of an administered society in which the centralization of information about citizens is essential for social planning. Foucault, too, highlights the social role of medical knowledge in controlling populations and like Parsons emphasizes the diffuse nature of power relationships in modern society. Also, like Parsons, he sees the professions, especially the helping professions, playing a key role in inducing individuals to comply with 'normal' social roles. For Foucault, modern societies are systems of organized surveillance with the catch being that individuals conduct the surveillance on themselves, having internalized 'professional' models of what is appropriate behaviour (White, 2002).

The theoretical space available in sociological writings makes it possible to understand the multidimensionality of health and health care even in the changing contexts. And further, the phrase 'sociology of health' is becoming more popular than 'medical sociology' or 'sociology of medicine' for its inherent broader perspective and emphasis on sociological understanding (see, Akram, 2012). According to Sarah Nettleton (1995: 1–2), 'the sociology of health and illness is not confined to the narrow domain of the formal institutions of medicine. It is concerned with all those aspects of contemporary social life which impinge upon well-being throughout the life course'. Hence, she prefers the phrase 'sociology of health' over any other nomenclature such as 'sociology of medicine' or 'medical sociology' for this branch of sociology. Sol Levine (1987) strongly recommends that sociology of health is more accurate and appropriate designation for this section. According to Levine, 'it is interesting, too, that many of us who are quite critical of physicians and of medical sociology, in general, have been willing to retain the designation of our section and of our own professional identity as that of medical sociology with its more prestigious, if not exotic, overtones, instead of using what would really be a more appropriate and accurate designation of the section, the 'Sociology of Health'' (1987: 1–2).

Stacey and Homans also state that sociology of health and illness is more appropriate for this section of sociology than sociology of medicine. This section can be concluded quoting Stacey and Homans (1978: 295), 'While most sociologists have interpreted medicine in a broad sense to mean all those matters to do with health and illness, the phrase 'sociology of medicine' does imply a particular connection with the medical profession. The contribution of sociology must be with the whole range of knowledge, belief, feeling, organization, institutions, associated with health, and illness and thus connected with the whole range of workers, professionals, semi-professionals, para-professional, unpaid workers, and others who are involved in the health industry, including the patients in that industry'.

Sociology in India

The teaching of sociology as an academic discipline started at the Bombay University with Patrick Geddes joining as professor of civics and sociology in 1919. Geddes was succeeded by G.S. Ghurye. Another important centre for the early growth of teaching and research in sociology has been Lucknow University, where the pioneering role was played by Radha Kamal Mukerji, D.P. Mukerji, and D.N. Mazumdar (Singh, 2004). Indian sociology, in the early post-independence era, witnessed five important features: (i) professionalization of sociology; (ii) emergence of new institutional support for its teaching and support; (iii) beginning of specialization in research; (iv) methodological consciousness; and (v) emphasis on social relevance in terms of development planning and social reconstruction. Amidst these phases of professionalization, institutionalization, and differentiation, the need of Indianization of western sociological concepts and methods also attracted great attention.

The decade of 1950s, in Indian sociology, witnessed a proliferation in the studies of Indian village and it was followed by studies of tribe, caste, family, and religion. Sociology in India, in the succeeding years, witnessed two developments: contact with western sociologists and increased focus of the government towards planned social and economic change. Community development, population and health, social movement, democratic institutions, land reforms, scheduled castes and tribes, and various professions, such as law and medicine, attracted the attention of students and teachers of sociology during this period. In this period, many specialized branches of sociology find their origin. Four theoretical orientations prevalent over the period can be identified as: (i) philosophical, (ii) culturological, (iii) structural-theoretic, and (iv) dialectical-historic. Yogendra Singh (2004) summarizes the specific developments of the period: 'the early beginners of Indian sociology pioneered the vision of sociology and social science as having a historical-civilizational anchorage; they felt acutely uneasy in accepting the positivistic, utilitarian, and the general evolutionary constructions and premises of the western sociology; and they consistently introduced the perspectives of historicity, culture, and values in the formulation of sociological concepts and their theoretical underpinnings' (2004: 145).

Sociology of Health in India

Aneeta Minocha (*nee* Ahluwalia) wrote a trend report in 1974 entitled 'Sociology of Medicine: A Trend Report' (Minocha, 1974) which was part of an ambitious project to carry out a survey of research done so far in the field of social sciences including sociology. Minocha states that 'sociology of medicine' is a new development in India and it is difficult, if not premature, to identify the trends in research done in the field so far. According to Minocha, the sociologist generally sees the field of medicine in two main aspects: (a) as a cultural complex, that is, a complex of material objects, tools, techniques, knowledge, ideas, and values and (b) as a part of social structure and organization, that is, a network of relations between groups, classes, and categories of persons. In both these aspects, sociology is interested in medicine just as it is interested in other aspects of social life such as religion or economy. This trend report was the first systematic attempt to identify and analyse the sociological (along with some anthropological) writings related to sociology of health (also identified as sociology of medicine). Minocha presented a selective bibliography of most of the works accessible to her without making any distinction between sociological and anthropological writings. Her own work related to heterogeneity and pluralism in traditional and modern systems of medicine is a great contribution towards development of sociology of health in India.

According to Mehta (1982), the topics identified by Minocha were promoted by the foreign sociologists and anthropologists who carried out studies on rural India. Such studies had western paradigms, models, and concepts. During the 1970s, there was an alarm raised against these and a plea was given for Indianization of the studies in terms of orientation, approach, and value relevance. Mehta divides the studies conducted on themes related to health, disease, and medicine in India in two categories: (a) providers of health and medical care, and (b) consumers of health and medical care. However, Mehta is obsessed with the term 'medical' and did not talk about a more general concept, 'health'. He does not seem to be impressed with the Alma Ata Declaration (1978) or a broad definition of health as given by World Health Organization (WHO).

In the last 20 years, sociology of health has grown a lot both at global level and in Indian context. In this period, sociology of health (very often medical sociology) became part of curriculum of many universities in India. Indian Sociological Society—the association of teachers and professional related to sociology—is having now a separate Research Committee for studying issues related to health and population. This research committee is doing a lot in giving platform to the research conducted at university and college level. The state level and regional associations are also making significant contribution in promoting sociology of health.

The beginning of National Family Health Surveys (NFHS) provided huge base line data related to household and health patterns. The human development and the social development reports significantly highlighted role of health in development. The health and population related periodic data provided by the National Sample Survey Organization (NSSO) is also enriching the secondary data base for sociologists. The period also witnessed large-scale, macro-level, and micro-level studies funded by various internal and external funding agencies. Developments related to health and health care and especially the national policies on health and population (often induced by global agencies such as United Nations, World Bank, and WHO) widened the interest within sociology of health. The increasing emphasis on 'social determinants of health' also made sociological research very relevant.

Phases of Sociology of Health in India

Every discipline or sub-discipline passes through certain phases in its move towards maturity and independence. Three phases of development of 'sociology of health' in India have been proposed by the present author on the basis of developments within and outside the discipline. The proposed phases are tentative and meant for reflecting the nature and scope of the sub-discipline only. (It should be acknowledged here that this classification was originally presented in a paper on 'Development of Sociology of Health In India: Phases, Paradigms and Future' during the XVII ISA World Congress of Sociology organized by International Sociological Association, held at Gothenburg, Sweden (11–17 July 2010). The detailed paper is published in *Salute e Società* (English), XI–2, 2012.89–115). Only some of the arguments are presented here.

The first phase started after independence (1947) and continued till imposition of political emergency (1975–76) in India. This phase witnessed lack of proper health infrastructure, high fertility and mortality, and limited interaction between sociologist and health institutions. The community development programme (CDP), establishment of primary health care centres and, lately, population control were the important driving forces of the government. The extreme steps for controlling population during the emergency period (late 1970s) attracted great number of sociologists towards population and health relations. The phase also witnessed impact of British and US sociology. The important areas of interest for sociologist were: types of medicine such as traditional, indigenous, urban, folk, and ethnic; medical pluralism; health system and sub-systems; doctor-patient relations; nursing staff and medical profession; health behaviour, culture, beliefs, and practices; and disease, treatment and illness patterns. The phase was dominated by the structural-functionalists, the interactionists, and the behaviourists in terms of theoretical perspectives and approaches.

The second phase started after the Alma Ata Declaration (1978) and continued till establishment of National AIDS Control Organization (NACO) in 1992 and was dominated by themes of health for all, family planning, poverty and malnutrition, health of children and aged, reproductive and adolescent health, etc. The Alma Ata Declaration had given new vision to health policies and programmes. The National Health Policy was formed in 1983 to make the architectural corrections in health care system. The Universal Immunization Programme (UIP) was launched in 1985 to provide universal coverage to infants and pregnant women. Fertility, mortality, declining sex ratio, environment and ecological concerns, and social and sustainable development were the other important topics that attracted health sociologists in that phase.

The phase witnessed inclusion of demographic and ecological perspectives within sociology of health. Besides structural-functionalism, interactionism, and behaviourism, the phase also witnessed the conflict and the phenomenological perspectives in various writings.

The third phase can be identified with the establishment of NACO in 1992 since the period witnessed growth of empirical and even social epidemiological studies of sexually transmitted diseases (STDs), AIDS, and reproductive tract infections (RTIs) among various occupational groups (truck drivers, cleaners, labourers, sex workers) and communities (tribal, rural, urban) along with issues related to health care, especially reproductive health and medical ethics. The phase witnessed launch of reproductive and child health programmes as well as National Rural Health Mission (NRHM). Some of the emerging and contemporary issues continuously drawing the attention of health sociologists in the new millennium are the Millennium Development Goals (MDGs); health-disparity (including gender-disparity) and impacts of globalization; health as basic human right of marginalized groups; health expenditure, funding, and insurance; privatization of health; and public-private partnership. The phase is witnessing flood of data-based surveys and empirical studies. Along with the social epidemiological studies, phenomenological, ethnomethodological, ethnographic, and narrative studies are also becoming quite popular.

Future of Sociology of Health in India

According to WHO, a good health system delivers quality services to all people, when and where they need them. Development of a well-integrated health system is a long-term and enduring process. The task is more challenging for India because of its colonial past. The Bhore Committee had submitted its recommendation way back in 1946 and these formed the basis for the establishment of organizations of basic health services in India. Since then, a good number of committees submitted their reports for the improvement of health services, and the five-year plans documented specific targets to improve health services. The primary health centres and sub-centres and the community development programmes were the backbone of health initiative in India in the first three decades after independence. The national health policies and subsequent reforms and missions are responding to the felt need of people of India. Sociology of health in India, under these circumstances, is an important sub-discipline of sociology. With the increasing realization of importance of health and widening dimensions of the notion of health, the scope of sociology of health is bound to increase.

India is on the verge of demographic transition. It is also witnessing the initial elements of epidemiological transition. Several initiatives related to promotion of health and combating disease have been taken in the last two decades in India. The first policy on health came in India only in 1980s. Before that, we had the vertical programmes addressing to specific diseases. The NRHM is an important development of the first decade of this millennium. Now, National Urban Health Mission (NUHM) will be addressing the unmet needs of the urban (especially the deprived) population. Universal Health Coverage, in order to meet the economic needs of health treatment and health care, is about to arrive as well. The UN Commission on Social Determinants of Health has very well established the need of understanding the social determinants of health and disease. Policy and planning in health is witnessing important shifts because of privatization and globalization. India is yet to have a standard mechanism of monitoring the quality of various service providers at national or state level. The government has very little effective presence in regulating the health-economics or even drug prices since these are mostly determined by the providers/manufacturers. Thus, there are challenges that the nation needs to address.

Sociology of health is one discipline that can address most of such issues. In United States, European countries, and other parts of developed world, understanding issues related to medical as well as non-medical dimensions of health is playing a crucial role in combating the specific health challenges, and sociology of health is playing an important role in that. In India, sociology of health is maturing; it has started to leap forward and, I am sure, will be able to address the challenges in coming future.

Science and technology is the driving force of the present age. Global movement and technological invention is influencing the basic institutions of the society, and these are also resulting into commodification of human body and mind. Hence, a huge impact will be the change in the health requirements of human bodies. Some of the interventions that need great social understanding are new innovations in transplant surgery, heart bypass, artificial organs, ventilator assistance, renal dialysis, and various other ways of prolonging the life of a dying patient. The issues related to cloning and mercy killing have great sociological and ethical dimensions. The emergence of new social practices such as surrogate mother, hired womb, and live-in relations is bound to have new health concerns. In future, it will be the duty of health sociologists to simplify the issues through sound sociological and theoretical knowledge.

The biomedical model of health is still the dominant model of health in India. Government has started to give importance to the conventional and traditional systems of therapy through its organized effort of promoting AYUSH. But much remains in promoting the social and the preventive models to the extent that they can start complementing the biomedical model. In country like India, where health and disease are directly related to quality of life especially food, water, nutrition, hygienic living conditions, etc., people at younger age need to be educated to spend more on basic health goods such as nutrition, food, and sanitation, so that they are not compelled to spend more on treatment of disease at a later stage. This will help in building sustainable lifestyle. Education (especially of the parents) alone can cause great pre-mature mortality differentials.

The author believes that the concept of primary health care as envisaged by the Alma Ata Declaration (1978) has been neither understood properly in India nor implemented at grass roots level. The notion of primary health care suggests a mechanism to prevent diseases from occurring and further providing local and accessible solutions for the treatment. However, the primary health centres (PHCs) that we have in most of the states in India are not based on such principles and the states are struggling hard to provide sufficient staff and professionals at that level. Sociology of health can provide the basic principles for meeting such needs.

However, following western notions blindly will not serve the purpose. There is a need to methodologically address the health-related issues of Indian population. The study of prevailing disease patterns and their socio-cultural causation needs special attention. The 'public health' component of health is almost missing in India. An absolute medicalization of health is a big threat for the society. A comprehensive paradigm, taking into consideration the grounded realities and spatial/social variation, is the need of the hour. The author has used the concept of dehealthism to understand some of the ongoing processes in India. We need to find out many more under currents and practices, which are preventing the attainment of the goal of 'health for all'. Let us hope, sociology of health and disease in India will come up to the expectation of its health-deprived population.

References

Akram, M. (2012). 'Development of Sociology of Health: A Review of the Contexts and Phases, Themes and Future in India', *Salute e Società (Sociology and Sociology of Health: A Round Trip)*, XI–2 (English) 89–115.

Clarke, J. (1981). 'A Multiple Paradigm Approach to the Sociology of Medicine, Health and Illness', *Sociology of Health and Illness*, 3 (1): 89–103.

Cockerham, W.C. (2007). *Social Causes of Health and Disease*, USA: Polity Publication.

Cockerham, W.C. and Ritchey, F.J. (1997). *Dictionary of Medical Sociology*, London: Greenwood Press.

De Maio, F. (2010). *Health and Social Theory*, New York: Palgrave Macmillan.

Foucault, M. (1973). *The Birth of Clinic*, First published by Tavistock Publications Limited in 1973, First published in Routledge Classics in 2003, Oxon.

Gerhardt, U. (1989). *Ideas about Illness: An Intellectual and Political History of Medical Sociology*, Basingstoke: Macmillan.

Larkin, M. (2011). *Social Aspects of Health, Illness and Healthcare*, New York: Open University Press.

Levine, S. (1987). 'The Changing Terrains in Medical Sociology: Emergent Concerns with Quality of Life', *Journal of Health and Social Behaviour*, 28 (March): 1–6.

Lupton, D. (2003). *Medicine as Culture; Illness, Disease and the Body in Western Societies*, Second Edition, London: Sage Publications.

Mechanic, D. (1978). *Medical Sociology*, New York: The Free Press.

Mehta, S.R. (1982). 'Sociology of Health and Medical Care: Research Needs and Challenges', in Nayar, P.K.B. (ed.), *Sociology of India* (pp. 301–328), New Delhi: B.R. Publishing Corp.

Minocha (Ahluwalia), Aneeta. (1974), 'Sociology of Medicine: A Trend Report', in M.N. Srinivas, M.S.A Rao, and A.M. Shah (eds.), *A Survey of Research in Sociology and Social Anthropology*, Vol. II (401–430). Bombay: Popular Prakashan.

Nettleton, S. (1995). *The Sociology of Health and Illness*, UK: Polity Press.

Raphael, D., Bryant, T. and Rioux, M. (eds.). (2006). *Staying Alive: Critical Perspectives on Health, Illness, and Health Care*, Toronto, Ontario: Canadian Scholars' Press Inc.

Scambler, G. (ed.). (1987). *Sociological Theory and Medical Sociology*, London: Tavistock Publications.

Singh, Y. (2004). *Ideology and Theory in Indian Sociology*, Jaipur: Rawat Publications.

Stacey, M. and Homans, H. (1978). 'The Sociology of Health and Illness: Its Present State, Future Prospect and Potential for Health Research', *Sociology*, 12(2): 281–307.

Straus, R. (1957). 'The Nature and Status of Medical Sociology', *American Sociological Review*, 22: 200–204.

Thomas, R.K. (2002). *Society and Health: Sociology for Health Professionals*, New York: Kluwer Academic Publishers.

Turner, B. (2006). *The Cambridge Dictionary of Sociology*, Cambridge: Cambridge University Press.

White, K. (2002). *An Introduction to the Sociology of Health and Illness*, London: Sage Publications

——. (2009). *An Introduction to the Sociology of Health and Illness*, second edition, London: Sage Publications.

Chapter Two

Social Medicine and Community Health

Social Medicine

In the nineteenth century, social medicine emerged as a movement to investigate medical problems in the light of social science. More than anyone else it was French physician Jules Guerin who introduced the term 'social medicine', and he urged his colleagues to help in creating a new society following the Revolution of 1848 (Cockerham and Ritchey, 1997). The idea of 'social medicine' spread throughout Europe and England after the First World War. The industrial revolution and the subsequent increase in poverty and disease among workers raised concerns about the effect of social processes on the health of the poor. According to Park (2009), social medicine is not a new branch of medicine but somewhat an extension of the public health idea reflecting the strong relationship between medicine and social sciences or a new orientation of medicine to the changing needs of man and society.

Cockerham and Ritchey (1997) have given an extensive definition of social medicine. According to them, 'social medicine is a broad field embracing the social and behavioral sciences, along with the humanities in the analysis of the relationship between society, health and medicine. Subject areas include but are not limited to examining the role of medicine as a social institution; the social effects of medical knowledge; social origins of health and disease morbidity; health lifestyles; social and political philosophies underlying health care delivery systems; societal norms, values and ethics pertaining to medical practice; the culture of medicine and health; and the social history of medicine. The goal of social medicine is to produce knowledge enabling health practitioners and policy makers to make informed and effective decisions reflecting the social and cultural realities of the people they serve' (Cockerham and Ritchey, 1997: 119). The field of social medicine seeks to understand how social and economic conditions impact health, disease, and the practice of medicine and foster conditions in which this understanding can lead to a healthier society.

According to Park (2009: 44), social medicine is 'the study of a man as a social being in his total environment'. It is concerned with all the factors affecting the distribution of health and ill health in populations including the use of health services. Webster (1986) (as quoted in Sheaff, 2005: 119) says that 'social medicine is medical science in relation to groups of human beings … . It is not merely or mainly concerned with the prevention and elimination of sickness, but is also concerned with the study of all social agencies which promote or impair the fullest realization of biologically and socially valuable human capacities. It includes the application to problems of health and disease of sociological concepts and methods'.

White (2006), referring to Engels and Virchow, explains that disease is the product of the prevailing social conditions. Engels and Virchow argued that it was the social environment of developing capitalism that caused the great diseases of the eighteenth and nineteenth centuries—cholera and typhoid, tuberculosis and diphtheria. In their analyses the overcrowding of the new industrial cities, the development of slums, and the new factory organization of labour caused these diseases. Rather than examine the individual's body and search for bacteriological explanations of disease, this model identified the social environment as the source of sickness and ill health and suggested cleaning up the slums, keeping the water fresh and enforcing the hygienic production of foodstuffs. Historical epidemiology supports the argument that social reform rather than scientific medicine brought about the transformation in people's standards of health (White, 2006).

According to Park (2009: 44), 'the report on royal commission on medical education, 1968 (also known as Todd Report), for the first time, uses the term 'community medicine' instead of 'social medicine' and defined it in terms which embraced social medicine but went beyond it by giving greater emphasis to the organizational and administrative aspects than the academic social medicine in the past. This gave a blow to the further development of social medicine which had tended in many countries to be displaced by the newer term community medicine'.

Community Health

McKenzie, Pinger, and Kotecki (2005: 5), in their book *An Introduction to Community Health,* comment that 'community health refers to the health status of a defined group of people and the actions and conditions, both private and public (governmental), to promote, protect, and preserve their health. For example, the health status of the people of Muncie, Indiana and the private and public actions taken to promote, protect, and preserve the health of these people, would constitute community health'. 'Community health assesses the health requirements of a whole community and makes provisions to meet its health needs, to carry out research in community health, and to organize health education for all' (Mishra, 2007: 37). In order to perform the assigned social roles in society or in a group, functionalists regard community health as an important aspect for keeping the members of society in a healthy state or condition. They believe that community health may contribute in the process of integration of the society.

The EURO symposium in 1966 defined community health as including 'all the personnel and environmental services in any human community, irrespective of such services were public or private ones'. In some instances community health is used as a synonym for 'environmental health' and is also used to refer to 'community health care' (Park, 2009).

Factors Affecting Community Health

According to McKenzie, Pinger, and Kotecki (2005), there are many factors that affect the health of a community. As a result, the health status of each community is different. These factors may be social and/or cultural (religious, political, economic, etc.) or physical. They also include the ability of the community to organize and work together as a whole as well as the individual behaviours of those in the community. These factors, identified by McKenzie, Pinger, and Kotecki, are briefly presented here:

Social and Cultural Factors

Social factors are those that arise from the interaction of individuals or groups within the community. For example, people who live in urban communities, where life is fast-paced, experience higher rates of stress-related illnesses than those who live in rural communities, where life is slower. On the other hand, those in rural areas may not have access to the same quality or selection of health care (i.e., providers, hospitals, or medical specialists) that is available to those who live in urban communities. Cultural factors arise from guidelines (both explicit and implicit) that individuals inherit from being a part of a particular society. Culture teaches us what to fear, what to respect, what to value, and what to regard as relevant in our lives.

Beliefs, Traditions, and Prejudices

The health of the community can also be affected by beliefs, traditions, and prejudices of community members. The beliefs of those in a community about such specific health behaviours as exercise and smoking can influence policy makers on whether or not they will spend money on bike trails and no-smoking ordinances. The traditions of specific ethnic groups can influence the types of food, restaurants, retail outlets, and services available in a community. Prejudices of one specific ethnic or racial group against another can result in acts of violence and crime. Racial and ethnic disparities will continue to put certain groups, such as Black Americans or certain religious groups, at greater risk.

Social Norms

Cigarette smoking is a good example to understand how it has effects on health of the community. During the 1940s, 1950s, and 1960s, it was socially acceptable to smoke in most settings. As a matter of fact, in 1960, 53 per cent of American men and 32 per cent of American women smoked. Thus, in 1960 it was socially acceptable to be a smoker, especially for a male. Now, early in the twenty-first century, those percentages have dropped to 25.2 per cent (for males) and 20.7 per cent (for females), and in most public places it has become socially unacceptable to smoke. The law suits against tobacco companies by both the state attorneys general and private citizens provide further evidence that smoking has fallen from social acceptability. Because of this change in the social norm, there is less second-hand smoke in many public places, and in turn the health of the community has improved. Unlike smoking, alcohol consumption represents a continuing negative social norm in America, especially on college campuses. The normal expectation seems to be that drinking is fun (and almost everyone wants to have fun). Despite the fact that most college students are too young to drink legally, 85 per cent to 90 per cent of college students drink. It seems fairly obvious that the American alcoholic beverage industry has influenced our social norms.

Socio-economic Status

The gap in health status and mortality between those commanding and those who lack economic power and social resources continues to widen in United States and Western Europe. This reflects the relationship between people's socio-economic position as consumers and employers or employees and their social, biological, and mental well-being. That is, those in the community with the lowest socio-economic status also have the poorest health and the most difficulty in gaining access to health care. The point of entry into the health care system for most Americans is the family doctor. The economically disadvantaged seldom have a family doctor. For them, the point of entry is the local hospital emergency room. In addition to health care access, higher incomes enable people to afford better housing, live in safer neighbourhoods, and increase the opportunity to engage in health promoting behaviours.

Religion

Religion can affect a community's health positively or negatively. There are number of religions which have taken a position on health care. For example, some religious communities prohibit certain foods. For example, Kosher dietary regulations permit Jews to eat the meat only of animals that chew cud and have cloven hooves and the flesh only of fish that have both gills and scales, while still others, such as the Native American Church of the Morning Star, use peyote, a hallucinogen, as a sacrament. Still others limit the type of medical treatment their members may receive. Some religious communities actively address moral and ethical issues such as abortion, premarital intercourse, and homosexuality. Some do not permit immunizations; others do not permit their members to be treated by physicians. Still other religions teach health-promoting codes of living to their members.

Economy

The health of a community is also affected by national and local economies through reductions in health and social services. An economic downturn means lower tax revenues (fewer tax dollars) and fewer contributions to charitable groups. Such actions will result in fewer dollars being available for programmes such as welfare, food stamps, community health care, and other community services. With less money, these agencies often must alter their eligibility guidelines, thereby restricting aid to only the neediest individuals. Obviously, many people who had been eligible for assistance before the economic downturn become ineligible. Employers usually find it increasingly difficult to provide health benefits for their employees as their income drops. Those who are unemployed and underemployed face poverty and deteriorating health. Thus, the growing effect of an economic downturn significantly affects the health of the community.

Politics

Those who happen to be in political office, either nationally or locally, can improve or make vulnerable the health of their community by the decisions they make. In the most general terms, the argument is over greater or lesser governmental participation in health issues. For example, there has been a long-standing discussion in the United States on the extent to which the government should involve itself in health care. Historically, democrats have been in favour of such action, while republicans have been against it. However, as the cost of health care continues to grow, both democrats and republicans see the need for some kind of increased regulation. Local politicians also influence the health of their communities each time they vote on health-related measures brought before them.

Physical Factors

Physical factors include the influences of geography, the environment, community size, and industrial development.

(a) Geography

A community's health problems can be directly influenced by its altitude, latitude, and climate. In tropical countries where warm, humid temperatures and rain prevail throughout the year, parasitic and infectious diseases are a leading community health problem. In many tropical countries, survival from these diseases is made more difficult because poor soil conditions result in inadequate food production and malnutrition. In temperate climates with fewer parasitic and infectious diseases and a more than adequate food supply, obesity and heart disease are important community health problems.

(b) Environment

The quality of our environment is directly related to the quality of our stewardship over it. Many experts believe that if we continue to allow uncontrolled population growth and continue to deplete non-renewable natural resources, succeeding generations will inhabit communities that are less desirable than ours. Many feel that we must accept responsibility for this stewardship and drastically reduce the rate at which we foul the soil, water, and air.

(c) Community size

Community size is the one of the important factor that affects community health. Community size can impact both positively and negatively on that community health. The larger the community size, the greater the range of health problems and the greater will be its number of health resources. For example, larger communities have more health professionals and better health facilities than smaller communities. These resources are often needed because communicable diseases can spread more quickly, and environmental problems are often more severe in densely populated areas. For example, the amount of garbage generated by approximately 8 million people in New York City is many times greater than the amount generated by the entire state of Wyoming, with its population of about 5,01,000.

Industrial Development

Industrial development can have either positive or negative effects on the health status of a community. Industrial development provides a community with more resources for community health programmes, but it may bring with it environmental pollution and occupational illnesses. Communities that experience rapid industrial development must eventually regulate the way in which industries (i) obtain raw materials, (ii) discharge by-products, (iii) dispose of wastes, (iv) treat and protect their employees, and (v) clean up environmental accidents. Unfortunately, many of these laws are usually passed only after these communities have suffered significant reductions in the quality of their life and health.

References

Cockerham, W.C. and Ritchey, F.J. (1997). *Dictionary of Medical Sociology*, London: Greenwood Press.

McKenzie, J.F., Pinger, R.R. and Kotecki, J.E. (2005). *An Introduction to Community Health*, London: Jones and Bartlett Publishers.

Mishra, R.P. (2007). *Geography of Health*, Delhi: Concept Publications.

Park, K. (2009). *Preventive and Social Medicine* 20th edition, Jabalpur: Banarsidas Bhanot.

Webster, C. (1986). 'The Origins of Social Medicine in Britain', *Bulletin of the Society for the Social History of Medicine*, 38: 52–55 as cited in Sheaff, M. (2005). *Sociology and Health Care*, New York: Open University Press.

White, K. (2006). *The Sage Dictionary of Health and Society*, Delhi: Sage Publications.

CHAPTER THREE

Sociological Perspectives on Health

Gabe, Bury, and Elson in their book *Key Concepts in Medical Sociology,* explain the importance of sociological perspective while studying health and illness. According to them, 'Sociology can relate to health and illness in two different ways. On the one hand, a sociological perspective can be applied to the experience and social distribution of health and health disorders and to the institutions through which care and cure are provided. In this sense, medical sociology can have an applied orientation to understanding and improving health and can be seen as one of many disciplines that might appropriately be studied by providers of health care. On the other hand, the sociological study of health, illness, and institutions of health care can stand alongside analysis of other significant social experiences and institutions, as a means of understanding the society under study. Thus, medical sociology is also a theoretically orientated field, committed to explaining large-scale social transformations and their implications, as well as interactions in everyday settings, as these are expressed in health and illness' (Gabe, Bury, and Elson, 2004: ix).

From 1946 to 1951, the new field of medical sociology became completely an applied area of research. The link between medical sociology and sociological theory was crucial to the sub-discipline because theory binds medical sociology to the larger discipline of sociology more extensively than any other aspect of the sociological enterprise (Cockerham, 2010). In fact, it was only in the last third of the twentieth century) that the contribution of the sociological perspective to the study of health and health care came to be appreciated. There have been three dominant theoretical perspectives in the history of medical sociology/sociology of health and illness: functionalism, conflict, and symbolic interactionism.

Functional Perspective

The first approach to be examined is functionalism, which contends that health and illness reflect the level of social normality rather than physical normality characterizing an individual (Parsons, 1972). This theoretical approach is based on an analogy between the society and a biological organism. Just as the body consists of different but interrelated and interdependent parts, similarly society consists of a number of different systems and sub-systems. These different parts achieve a unity in so far as they function to sustain the whole. Therefore, functionalism is less concerned with the individual actions and his or her aims, beliefs, and consciousness, rather with how these actions and beliefs, etc., function to maintain the system as a whole (Barry and Yuill, 2002).

According to Cockerham (2010), a crucial event occurred in 1951 that oriented medical sociology towards theoretical concerns and initiated the establishment of its academic credentials. This was the publication of Talcott Parsons' book, *The Social System*, in which Parsons used the medical profession as a model; he analysed the needs of the system and expressed in the duties and reciprocal entitlements of both doctor and patient. For the doctor, the pattern variables of universalism, performance, or achievement, rather than ascription, specificity, and affective neutrality, were appropriate. The rights, obligations, and privileges of the sick role described the norms of being a patient. This ideal-type contract was what would, theoretically, identify medicine as functional in maintaining equilibrium in society and maintaining social order (Turner, 2006). Parsons' publication attracted great attention because he was thought to be charting a course for all of sociology. This book, providing a structural-functionalist model of society, contained Parsons' concept of the sick role. It was the first time a major sociological theorist included an analysis of the function of medicine in his view of society.

According to the functionalist approach, if society has to function as a stable system, it is necessary for its members to be healthy and also to contribute to their society's equilibrium. Consequently, sickness is viewed as a form of deviant behaviour that must be controlled by society. This view was initially set forth by Parsons (1951) in his concept of the sick role. The sick role is a shared set of cultural norms that legitimates deviant behaviour caused by the illness and channels the individual into the health care system. Tischler (2011) has mentioned the following four components of Parsons' notion of sick role:

1. The sick person is excused from normal social roles/responsibilities except to the extent that he or she is supposed to do whatever is necessary to get well.
2. The sick person is not held responsible for his or her condition and is not expected to recover by an act of will.
3. The sick person must recognize that being ill is undesirable and must want to recover.
4. The sick person is obligated to seek medical care and cooperate with the advice of the designated experts, notably the physicians. In this sense, although sick people are not blamed for their illnesses, they must work towards regaining their health.

The concept of sick role is used to analyse sickness as a social role, not merely as a biological entity and physical experience. Taking these characteristics into consideration, Parsons believed that illness is dysfunctional for both individuals and the larger society (Kendall, 2011; Tischler, 2011). Thus, according to functionalist perspective, the sick role exempts the patient from routine activities for a period of time, and assumes that the individual will seek appropriate medical attention and get well as soon as possible. Those people taking on the sick role do so only if they agree to comply with the regime given by the medical practitioner and if they are committed to getting well as soon as possible' (Cockerham, 2010; Cockerham, 2007; Barry and Yuill, 2002).

Thus, Parsons' model of the sick role is an 'ideal type', characterizing abstract generalization and exaggeration of empirical reality. And hence, sick people do not always become patients and not all patients are sick.

The functionalist perspective is a consensual approach to understanding society, which also assumes that the latent or hidden functions of everyday activities have significance for maintaining the system as a whole. In relation to something as simple as eating, Lupton (1996: 8) argues that the 'function' of food can be seen in broader terms than just as nutritional intake. A functionalist perspective serves to highlight the way in which 'food practices serve to support co-operative behaviour or structures of kinship in small groups'. Lupton has also argued that the meal is a way of illustrating the culture of a specific society in terms of the order in which food is served (savoury then sweet) and the mixing of food types and temperatures.

According to Parsons, 'it is important for the society to maintain social control over the people who enter into the sick role. Physicians are empowered to determine who may enter this role and when patients are ready to exit it. Because physicians spend many years in training and have specialized knowledge regarding illness, disease, and their treatment, they are certified by the society to be 'gatekeepers' of the sick role. When patients seek the advice of a physician, they enter into the patient-physician relationship, which does not contain equal powers for both parties. The patient is expected to follow the 'doctor's orders' by adhering to a treatment regime, recovering from the malady, and returning to a normal routine as soon as possible' (Kendall, 2011: 603). 'On the other hand, when patients arrive at the medical encounter, they are expected to surrender their medical knowledge and be guided by the medical 'experts'' (Gabe, Bury, and Elson, 2004: 64).

Kendall further states, 'Parsons' analysis of the sick role was path breaking when it was introduced. Some social analysts believe that Parsons made a major contribution to our knowledge of how society explains illness-related behaviour and how physicians have attained their gatekeeper status. In contrast, other analysts believe that the sick role model does not take into account racial-ethnic, class, and gender variations in the ways that people view illness and interpret this role. For example, this model does not take into account the fact that many individuals in the working class may choose not to accept the sick role unless they are seriously ill—because they cannot afford to miss time from work and lose a portion of their earnings' (Kendall, 2011). Despite this, structural functionalism, with its emphasis on value consensus, social order, stability, and functional processes at the macro level of society, had a short-lived period as the leading theoretical paradigm in medical sociology. In relation to the sick role, for example, it has been suggested that Parsons overlooked the potential for conflict between the patient and the practitioner and that he misguidedly assumed that the practitioner would always act in the best interests of the patient (Cockerham, 2007).

A direct connection between culture and health was articulated by Malinowski who considered culture as a functional response to satisfy 'the organic and basic needs of man and of the race'. Malinowski defined culture as 'the integral whole' encompassing 'human ideas and crafts, beliefs and customs … . A vast apparatus, partly material, partly human and partly spiritual by which man is able to cope with the concrete specific problems that face him'. Malinowski saw those problems as human 'needs' that promoted 'cultural responses'. These needs were metabolism, reproduction, bodily comforts, safety, movement growth, and health. However, in his view, health is implied in all the other six human needs in addition to the need for 'relief or removal of sickness or of pathological conditions'. He proposed 'hygiene' as the 'cultural response' to health. Hygiene involves all 'sanitary arrangements' in a community, 'native beliefs as to health and magical dangers', 'rules about exposure, extreme fatigue, the avoidance of dangers or accidents', and the 'never absent range of household remedies' (Cockerham, 2001: 25–26).

Citing references from different sources, Raphael, Bryant, and Rioux (2006) say that Parsons was more theoretical than empirical. According to them, 'Parsons' conceptualization came under significant criticism for how it masks the variability in the temporary or legitimate nature of different illnesses, and the diversity in the actual behaviour of sick individuals and of their providers. Twaddle (1969), for example, claimed that there are multiple configurations of the sick role of which Parsons is but one. Mechanic and Volkart (1960) also noted how Parsons' description was most relevant to acute illnesses, and not the increasingly prevalent chronic illnesses and disabilities that would entail a permanent role status. With respect to the provider's role, Szasz and Hollender (1956) refined Parsons' work by elaborating different doctor-patient models arising from different types of illness. The first matched patient passivity and physician assertiveness—most akin to Parsons' sick role—as the most common reaction to acute illness. The second was characterized by physician guidance and patient cooperation where a less acute illness was involved. The third model was characterized by physicians providing advice on a treatment plan that patients had most of the responsibility to implement; this last case was most relevant for chronic illnesses and certain forms of disability' (Raphael, Bryant, and Rioux, 2006: 37–38).

French sociologist Emile Durkheim emphasized the importance of macro-level social processes, structures, norms, and values (which he called 'social facts'), which are external to individuals and were capable of exerting external constraints on the behaviour of individuals causing them to act in a particular way, and integrated them into the larger society. People were depicted as constrained in exercising free will by the social order. Durkheim's only work that had a direct application to medical sociology is his theory of 'suicide' in which the act of taking one's life was determined by the individual's ties to his or her community or society. This is seen in his typology of three major types of suicide: (1) egoistic (social detachment), (2) anomic (state of normlessness), and (3) altruistic (a normative demand for suicide) (Cockerham, 2007). The merit of his concept is that it shows the capability of the larger society to create stressful situations where people are forced to respond to conditions not of their own choosing. Thus, Durkheim helps us not only to understand the social facets of suicide, but also to recognize that macro-level social events (such as economic recessions) can affect health in a variety of ways through stress and that the effects of stress can be mitigated through social support.

Cockerham (2007) concludes that Durkheim also influenced the study of health professions in noting the transition from mechanical to organic social solidarity, with its emphasis on specialization, in the modern division of labour. The boldness in Durkheim's work is his insistence that social forces (social facts)—external to the individuals—have a direct control upon their behaviour and can affect their health and in some situations curtailing their lives. Durkheim's work attracted sociologists and maintains that society exists external to the individual to constitute a reality of its own having a strong capacity to influence individual social behaviour. Durkheim finally concludes by asserting that 'social reality does not pertain to material objects but is an awareness of social norms, attitudes and values that are real in the sense that they are standards of behaviour that everyone is expected to follow. Deviation from these standards can have serious consequences (i.e., social rejection, loss of companionship and perhaps death or prison), for the person who chooses to ignore them' (Cockerham, 2007: 26–27).

Conflict Perspective

Marxist theory takes us back to the concern with the structure of society, suggesting that it is the economic structure of any society that determines the social relations contained within that structure. It is the distribution of the ownership of the means of production that gives rise to specific patterns of class relations, which, crucially, in all societies are characterized by inequalities of power. It is argued by Marxists that social change is the product of changes in economic relationships. Marxism explains social phenomena as primarily determined by the economic structure of society (Choudhary, 2006). Conflict theory, with its roots in the work of Karl Marx, is based on the assumption that society is composed of various groups struggling for advantage, inequality is a basic feature of social life, and conflict is the major cause of social change.

Conflict theory, which is different from the functionalist approach, emphasizes on the social, economic, and political forces that affect health, disease and the health care delivery system of people in the society. 'Among the issues of concern to conflict theorists are the ability of all people to obtain health care; how race, class, and gender inequalities affect health and health care; power relationships between doctors and other health care workers; the dominance of the medical model of health care; and the role of profit in the health care system' (Kendall, 2011: 604). The sociologists looking at health from the conflict approach are concerned with the relation between health, illness, and social organization within a society and how their meanings and definitions are influenced by the economic activity. There are various entities in the field of health and medicine that are providing the health care services. The focus of conflict theorists in health is on the struggle or conflict between these various entities such as medical profession, drug companies, insurance companies, business communities, and others (Darulius and Kaminskas, 2007). Marx's perspective in conflict theory is seen in the rejection of the view expressed by structural functionalism that society is held together by shared norms and values.

Marxist tradition in the sociology of medicine specifically attempts to link diseases to structural, economic, and political developments. Conflict theory claims that true consensus does not exist; rather society's norms and values are those of the dominant elite and imposed by them on the less privileged to maintain their advantaged position. However, Max Weber adds that social inequality is not merely based on unequal distribution of money, property, and relationships to the means of production, but also on status and political influence. Since all social systems contain such inequality, conflict inevitably results and conflict, in turn, is responsible for social change. Conflict theory allows us to chart the manoeuvres of various entities, like the medical profession, insurance companies, drug companies, the business community, and the public, as they struggle to acquire, protect, or expand their interests against the existing government regulations and programmes and those under consideration. Other conflict approaches are connected more directly to classical Marxism by relying on class struggle to explain health policy outcomes and the disadvantages of the lower and working classes in capitalist medical systems where the emphasis is on profit (Cockerham, 2010). While a major focus of conflict theory in medical sociology is on the role of competing interests in health care delivery and policy, other interests concern the sources of illness and disability in work environments, working class health, differences in health lifestyles, and capitalist ideologies in the physician-patient relationship.

Marxist theory is used to question the naturalness of capitalist relations and to unmask the reality of what is fundamentally an exploitative relationship. This theoretical approach is representative of a structural analysis of society, less concerned with the micro elements and more concerned with the larger picture, the underlying factors that explain social, economic, and political relationships.

Marxist political economy of health needs to address how the diversity of capitalist societies relates to medicine, health, and illness. Under political economy perspective, good health in political terms is defined not only as a state of physical or emotional well-being but also as 'access to and control over the basic material and non-material resources that sustain and promote life at a high level of satisfaction', meaning that 'a key component of health is struggle' (Baer, Singer, and Johnsen, 1986: 95). For political economists, ill, aged, and physically disabled people are marginalized by society because they do not contribute to the production and consumption of commodities. Other marginalized groups, such as women, people from non-English-speaking backgrounds, non-Whites, the aged, the unemployed, and members of the working class, tend to endure greater social and economic disadvantage than those from privileged groups and have restricted access to health care services. According to Petersen and Waddell (1998), this restricted access to health care services results in poor health or illness for these groups. Though it is the responsibility of the health care service providers to ensure that the population remains healthy enough to contribute to the economic system as workers and consumers, they are unwilling to devote the resources for those who do not respond to treatment and who are unable to return to the labour market. Thus, medicine serves to continue social inequalities, the divide between the privileged and underprivileged, rather than improve them. Political economy writers comment on the 'cultural crisis of modern medicine', in which health care under capitalism is perceived as largely ineffective, overly expensive, under-regulated, and vastly inequitable.

According to Kendall (2011), among few industrialized nations, United States relies almost exclusively on the medical-industrial complex for health care delivery and does not have universal health coverage, which provides some level of access to medical treatment for all people. Consequently, access to high-quality medical care is linked to people's ability to pay and to their position within the class structure. Those who are affluent or have good medical insurance may receive high-quality, state-of-the-art care in the medical-industrial complex because of its elaborate technologies and treatments. However, people below the poverty level and those just above it have greater difficulty of gaining access to medical care. Referred to as the medically indigent, these individuals do not earn enough to afford private medical care but earn just enough money to keep them from qualifying for Medicaid. In the profit-oriented capitalist economy, these individuals are said to 'fall between the cracks' in the health care system. This obviously shows how the gap in socio-economic conditions results in profound gap in health status of the poor in the United States.

In a Marxist approach, the function of medicine is the maintenance of the capitalist system. The medical profession controls labour through its control of the sick certificate, while the theories of disease it develops and enforces individualize the causes of disease and ignore social factors, thus performing an ideological function in stabilizing the status quo. Medical knowledge and technology do not have a separate existence from capitalist social relations; rather they are the product of the capitalism (White, 2006). Marxists further argues that disease and treatment are the outcomes of a capitalist economic system. The key test in the Marxist tradition is F. Engels' *The Condition of Working Class in England* (1974). Engels argues that disease is the direct outcome of capitalist's pursuit of profit at the expense of safety. By safety means not industrial matters, but housing conditions and food quality. In the Marxist perspective, medicine plays both an economic and an ideological role in contemporary society, which can be summarized as follows:

(i) medicine is the object-centred rather than person-centred, treating the human beings as things,
(ii) disease is seen as a condition to be treated by chemical or electronic intervention to restore balance in the body, rather than the outcome of the social relationships,

(iii) health is defined as fitness to carry out social role, particularly, the ability to sell labour, and

(iv) medicine focuses on the individual and the individualistic conceptions of lifestyles.

Raphael, Bryant, and Rioux (2006) have directly applied Marxist concepts to the study of health and health care. In their focus on the labour process under capitalism, they argue that there is a contradiction between the search of profit and ensuring the safety of workers. That is, the capitalist mode of production actually produces disease or what some have referred to as the social production of disease hypothesis. This could be directly in terms of physical, chemical, or biological pathogens at the workplace or in terms of the stress or risks of accidents as a result of the increasing intensification and fragmentation of work and alienation from the work process. They argues, for example, that morbidity and mortality are higher among individuals doing routine types of work requiring low levels of skills than among individuals working in jobs that demand a large number of skills and which allow for some type of control over one's own work (Navarro, 1986: 123). According to Vicente Navarro (1976), the capitalist state's involvement in health care brings about three things: it reproduces the class structure, it reproduces individualist ideology, and it reproduces alienation. The first of these outcomes is realized via the hierarchies among health workers. In modern capitalist societies, doctors are usually middle-class men, whereas nurses and health auxiliaries are usually lower middle-class or working-class women. Thus, the structure of the biomedical hierarchy reproduces the existing class and gender divisions. With respect to ideology, state involvement in health care sustains ideas and practices which suggest that the causes of ill health reside within individuals and their behaviour. Biomedicine as it is practised in modern capitalist economies rarely focuses on the economic and political factors responsible for illness and disease. Finally, state involvement in health care reproduces alienation. One of the roots of alienation lies in divisions between those who govern and those who are governed, those who administer and those who are administered, and those who are experts and those who are the recipients of 'expertise'. In modern capitalist economies, doctors and other health professionals are the governors and experts. As a result, their clients may feel isolated from the means by which they might recover their health and well-being (Aggleton, 1990).

Despite the negative health impacts of capitalist society on the labour process, the driving down of wages and general economic inequality has also been shown to influence health. Although not explicitly employing a Marxist perspective, many studies of social class differences in health status employ a materialist perspective in the spirit of their arguments. One of the most famous is the 1982 Black report on inequalities in health, which addresses the persistence of class differences in health in Britain despite the supposed 'equal access to health services' following the introduction of the National Health Service (Raphael, Bryant, and Rioux, 2006).

According to many conflict theorists, problems in US health care delivery are rooted in the capitalist economy that views medicine as a commodity, which is produced and sold by the medical-industrial complex. The medical-industrial complex encompasses local physicians and hospitals as well as global health-related industries such as insurance companies and pharmaceutical and medical supply companies. They further made their commitment that physicians—who hold a legal monopoly over medicine—benefit from the existing structure because they can charge inflated fees. Similarly, clinics, pharmacies, laboratories, hospitals, supply manufacturers, insurance companies, and many other corporations derive excessive profits from the existing system of payment in medicine (Kendall, 2011). The conflict theorists in medical sociology did not deny the fact that modern health care system has played an important role in improving the health status of population but they focus on various inequities that are inherent in the system. Therefore from the conflict perspective, the inequality inherent in our society is responsible for the unequal access to medical care (Andersen and Taylor, 2011). Ivan Illich, using this perspective in his medical nemesis, argues that the medical establishments are not interested in curing the disease of the patient; rather, they are interested in perpetuating their own self-interest studies (Stolley, 2005).

Alienation is one of Marx's more famous theories where he attempts to illuminate the lived experiences of capitalism, highlighting the lack of control and self-realization in the labour process. Workers in capitalist society are alienated from the product, productive activity, himself, community, and also from their fellows who have a profound effect on workers health. Throughout his work, Marx himself powerfully comments on how alienation has a variety of debilitating effects on the health of the worker in capitalist society—which squanders human beings, living labour, more readily than any other mode of production, squandering not only flesh and blood, but nerves and brain as well. According to Marx, capitalism deforms basic human nature to labour. This results in the productive activity, which is a pleasurable and rewarding experience, becoming the source and cause of all that is wrong in life. This is alienation which Marx outlines as being: the fact that labour is external to the worker, that is, it does not belong to his intrinsic nature; that in his work, therefore, he does not affirm himself but denies himself, does not feel content but unhappy, and does not develop freely his physical and mental energy but mortifies his body and his mind. Therefore, the worker only feels himself outside his work, and in his work feels outside himself, the spontaneous activity of the human imagination, of the human brain and the human heart, operates on the individual independently of him ... it is the loss of self.

From the above passage, the effects of alienation on the worker on a variety of related and interweaving levels can be deduced: alienation can affect not only the worker's health physically and mentally in terms of exhausting the body and the concentration of the mind required to work, but also emotionally—a point developed in depth later—in terms of the frustrating, unfulfilling dehumanization that alienated labour brings about (Yuill, 2005). From the above it can be said that conflict theorists increase our awareness of inequalities of race, class, and gender as these issues influence people's access to health care. They also inform us about the problems associated with health care becoming 'big business'. However, some analysts believe that the conflict approach is unduly pessimistic about the gains that have been made in health status and longevity—gains that are at least partially due to large investments in research and treatment by the medical-industrial complex.

Despite all this, it can be said that the use of conflict theory in medical sociology has several limitations: (i) all health situations are not affected by the conflict in the society; (ii) people may suffer from disease or may not be healthy because of various reasons, which in anyway may not be linked with politics, class conflict, interest group competition, and others (Darulius and Kaminskas, 2007).

Symbolic Interaction Perspective

In contrast to Parsons' structural functionalism, symbolic interactionism is based on the principle that there is a fundamental difference between the subject matter of sociology and that of the natural sciences. While the study of the natural world deals with physical, inanimate objects, the subject matter of sociology consists of people whose actions are motivated by human consciousness. Symbolic interactionism is therefore concerned with how people see and understand the social world. In studying health, symbolic interactionists focus on the meanings that social actors give their illness or disease and how these affect people's self-concept and relationships with others (Kendall, 2011).

'Symbolic interaction is the first major theoretical perspective to challenge Parsons' structural functionalist theory in medical sociology, which is based largely on the work of George Herbert Mead and Herbert Blumer. Symbolic interaction maintained that social reality is constructed on a micro level by individuals interacting with one another on the basis of shared symbolic meanings. Human beings were seen to possess the capacity to think, define situations, and construct their behaviour on the basis of their definitions and interpretations' (Cockerham, 2010: 7). 'Symbolic interaction perspective focuses on how health, health care, and illness of individuals are influenced by meanings, definitions, and labels and how such meanings are learned through interaction with others and through media messages and portrays' (Knox, 2008: 37). According to Patrick McNeill (1990), symbolic interactionists believe that individuals actively construct understandings of themselves using the evidence that comes from their interactions with others. Some of these interactions may lead them to understand themselves as healthy. In contrast to biomedical and social positivist researchers, interactionists tend to focus on the more subjective aspects of health.

Symbolic interactionist perspective is concerned with how people see and understand the social world. Symbolic interactionists believe that man can create and develop new symbolic environments and communities that nurture the sick, develop their skill, and motivate their increased participation in the social scene. Symbolic interactionist's perspective on health and health care provides us with new insights on the social construction of illness and how health and illness cannot be strictly determined by medical criteria. They are in the opinion that we socially construct 'health' and 'illness' and how both should be treated. For example, some people explain disease by blaming it on those who are ill. If we attribute cancer to the acts of a person, we can assume that we will be immune to that disease if we do not engage in the same behaviour. Non-smokers who learn that a lung cancer victim had a two-pack-a-day habit feel comforted that they are unlikely to suffer the same fate. Similarly, victims of AIDS are often blamed for promiscuous sexual conduct or intravenous drug use, regardless of how they contracted HIV. In this case, the social definition of the illness leads to the stigmatization of individuals who suffer from the disease. Although biological characteristics provide objective criteria for determining medical conditions such as heart disease, tuberculosis, or cancer, there is also a subjective component to how illness is defined. This subjective component is very important when we look at conditions such as childhood hyperactivity, mental illness, alcoholism, drug abuse, cigarette smoking, and overeating, all of which have been medicalized (see Kendall, 2011; Mechanic, 1978).

'The major figures in early medical sociology working in the symbolic interactionist tradition were Anselm Strauss and Erving Goffman'(Cockerham, 2001: 7). Strauss made his own contributions to theory and methods in a number of areas, including influential work on 'social process of death and dying'; observation of the 'negotiated order' of hospital routine featuring a minimum of 'hard and fast' regulations and a maximum of 'innovation and improvization' in patient care, especially in emergency treatment (Strauss et al., 1963). The significance of this approach can be seen in relation to understanding health behaviour that appears to be irrational. Graham (1993) examined patterns of cigarette smoking among mothers who belong to low-income households. What is revealed is relatively high levels of spending on cigarettes in low-income households. What can be observed or assumed is that this behaviour might well indicate a degree of irrationality in that it contradicts dominant health messages about the dangers of smoking and diverts limited financial resources away from the family. Graham, however, favours a theoretical approach dependent upon the symbolic interactionism tradition of interpreting human behaviour in the context of people's own beliefs and meanings.

According to Cockerham and Ritchey (1997), symbolic interaction has had great influence on studies of mental patients and provides the foundation for labelling theory, a major approach to explain deviant behaviour. Cockerham (1978) regards Friedson's labelling theory as a closest equivalent of symbolic interactionism. According to this theory, sickness may be a biological state but illness is created and formed by human perceptions. The treatment of deviant depends upon the label attached to the health of deviant by the members of the society. However, labelling theory, despite its merits in accounting for the powerful and often lasting effects of social 'labels' placed by others on individuals, could not explain the cause of deviance (other than the reactions of other people), nor whether deviants themselves shared common characteristics such as poverty, stress, or social backgrounds relevant to their deviance.

Sociologists expanded their work in mental health during the late 1950s and 1960s to include not only studies of mental patients but also studies of stigma, stress, families coping with mental disorder, and other areas of practical and theoretical importance. One of the key symbolic interactionist theorists who contributed to the field of medical sociology is Canadian-born sociologist Erving Goffman (1922–82). Because of his interest in how individuals develop their identity through the way in which others view them, he undertook an in-depth observational study of patients' subjective experience in mental institutions. Erving Goffman's book *Asylums* (1961), a study of life in a mental hospital, sets forth his concept of 'total institutions' that has emerged as a significant theoretical statement in the general discipline of sociology. An abundant literature subsequently evolved, making the sociology of mental disorder a major subfield within medical sociology.

In his later work, *Stigma* (1963), Goffman examines what he refers to as the management of a spoiled identity. He describes three main forms of stigma: (1) abominations of the body in the form of physical deformities; (2) blemishes of character in the form of socially deviant behaviour; and (3) groups with minority status in society (Cockerham and Ritchey, 1997). A variant of symbolic interactionism following along these studies by Goffman is labelling theory, which posits that the impact of labelling a person as ill or deviant means that others will respond to him or her in accordance with that label, which will be very difficult to shed. Labelling theory and Goffman's conceptualization of stigma led to a confusion of studies on the stigmatizing features of various illnesses from leprosy to epilepsy as well as how stigma can change over time and vary significantly across cultures (Raphael, Bryant, and Rioux, 2006).

Using the framework of symbolic interactionism, various studies have been carried out in India within the field of medical sociology. Srivastava, as noted by Mehta (1982), carried out the study in a hospital to study the nature and patterns of interaction between the doctors, the patients, and the paramedical staff; and Mathur, as noted by Mehta, carried out a study on the interpersonal relations between various categories of medical staff and the patients themselves.

Finally, this can be said that symbolic interactionists also make us aware of the importance of communication between physicians and patients, including factors that may reduce effective medical treatment for some individuals. However, these approaches have been criticized for suggesting that few objective medical criteria exist for many illnesses and for overemphasizing micro-level issues without giving adequate recognition to macro-level issues such as the effects on health care of managed care, health maintenance organizations, and for-profit hospital chains.

References

Aggleton, P. (1990). *Health*, London: Routledge Publications.

Andersen, M.L. and Taylor, H.F. (2011). *Sociology: The Essentials*, sixth edition, USA: Wadsworth, Cengage Learning.

Baer, H., Singer, M. and Johnsen, J. (1986). 'Towards a Critical Medical Anthropology', *Social Science and Medicine*, 23: 95–98.

Barry, A.M. and Yuill, C. (2002). *Understanding Health: A Sociological Introduction*, London/Thousand Oaks/New Delhi: Sage Publications.

Choudhary, S.K. (2006). *Thinkers and Theories in Sociology: From Comte to Giddens*, Delhi: Gangandeep Publications.

Cockerham, W.C. (1978). *Medical Sociology*, USA: Prentice Hall Inc.

——. (ed.). (2001). *The Blackwell Companion to Medical Sociology*, Oxford, UK: Blackwell Publishers.

——. (2007). *Social Causes of Health and Disease*, USA: Polity Publication.

——. (ed.). (2010). *The New Blackwell Companion to Medical Sociology*, United Kingdom: Wiley-Blackwell.

Cockerham, W.C. and Ritchey, F.J. (1997). *Dictionary of Medical Sociology*, London: Sage Westport.

Darulius, Z. and Kaminskas, R. (2007). *Peculiarities of Medical Sociology: Application of Social Theories in Analyzing Health and Medicine*, Lithuania: Kunas University of Medicine.

Gabe, J., Bury, M. and Elson, M. (2004). *Key Concepts in Medical Sociology*, London: Sage Publications.

Goffman, E. (1961). *Asylums*, New York: Doubleday and Anchor.

——. (1963). *Stigma: Notes on the Management of Spoiled Identity*. Engelwood Cliffs: Prentice Hall.

Graham, H. (1993). *When Life's a Drag: Women, Smoking and Disadvantage*. London: HMSO.

Kendall, D. (2011). *Sociology in Our Times*, eighth edition, Wadsworth, CA, USA: Cengage Learning.

Knox, D. (2008). *Understanding Social Problem*, USA: Wordsworth Cengage.

Lupton, D. (1996). *The Imperative of Health: Public Health and the Regulated Body*, London: Sage Publications.

McNeill, P. (1990). *Health*, London: Routledge Publications.

Mechanic, D. (1978). *Medical Sociology*, New York: The Free Press.

Mechanic, D., and E.H. Volkart. (1960). 'Illness Behavior and Medical Diagnosis.' *Journal of Health and Human Behavior*, 1(2): 86–93.

Mehta, S.R. (1982). 'Sociology of Health and Medical Care: Research Needs and Challenges', in Nayar, P.K.B. (ed.), *Sociology of India* (pp. 301–328), New Delhi: B.R. Publishing Corp.

Navarro, V. (1976). *Medicine under Capitalism*. New York: Prodist.

——. (1986). *Crisis, Health and Medicine: A Social Critique*. London: Tavistock.

Parsons, T. (1951). *The Social System*, New York: Free Press.

——. (1972). 'Definitions of Health and Illness in the Light of American Values and Social Structure', in Jaco, E.G. (ed.), *Patients, Physicians, and Illness*, New York: McMillan Publications.

Petersen, A.R. and Waddell, C. (1998). *Health Matters: A Sociology of Illness, Prevention and Care*. Sydney: Allen and Unwin.

Raphael, D, Bryant, T. and Rioux, M. (ed.). (2006). *Staying Alive: Critical Perspectives on Health, Illness, and Health Care*, Toronto, Ontario: Canadian Scholars' Press Inc.

Stolley, K.S. (2005). *The Basics of Sociology*, USA: Greenwood Publishing Group.

Strauss, A., Schatzman, L., Ehrlich, D., Bucher, R. and Sabshin M. (1963). 'The Hospital and its Negotiated Order'. pp. 147–69 in E. Freidson (ed.), *The Hospital in Modern Society*. New York: Free Press.

Szasz, J., and M. Hollender. (1956). 'The Basic Models of the Doctor-Patient Relationship.' *Archives of Internal Medicine*, 97: 585–592.

Tischler, H.L. (2011). *Introduction to Sociology*, tenth edition, USA: Wadsworth, Cengage Learning.

Turner, B. (2006). *The Cambridge Dictionary of Sociology*, Cambridge: Cambridge University Press

Twaddle, A.C. (1969). 'Health Decisions and Sick Role Variations: An Exploration.' *Journal of Health and Social Behavior*, 10(2): 105–114.

White, K. (2006). *SAGE Dictionary of Health and Society*, New Delhi: Sage Publications.

Yuill, C. (2005). 'Marx: Capitalism, Alienation and Health', *Social Theory and Health*, 3, 126–143, Palgrave Macmillan Ltd. http://medicina.kmu.lt/0702/0702–04e.pdf

Chapter Four

Epidemiology and Social Epidemiology

The term epidemiology comes from the Greek words *epi*, meaning 'on or upon', *demos*, meaning 'people', and *logos*, meaning 'the study of'. Epidemiology can be translated into the phrase 'the study of that which is upon the people'. Epidemiology is the branch of medicine that refers to 'study of the causes, distribution and determinants of diseases and injuries; and the ways of controlling its spread in human populations' (Hang, 2008: 614; Hansen and Easthop, 2007: 16). 'The goal of epidemiology is to limit disease, injury, and death in a community by intervening to prevent or limit outbreaks or epidemics of disease and injury' (McKenzie, Pinger, and Kotecki, 2005: 61). According to Turner (2006), epidemiology is defined as the study of the patterning and determinants of the incidence and distribution of disease. Discipline of epidemiology is concerned with environmental factors—whether physical, biological, chemical, psychological, and social—that affect health and also considers the course and outcomes of disease in individuals and in groups.

Epidemiology is the study of the distribution and determinants of health-related states or events in specified populations, and the application of this study to the control of health problems. This definition of epidemiology includes several terms that reflect some of the important principles of the discipline. The Epidemiology Program Office, Atlanta, Georgia, has explained the principles of epidemiology in its literature titled, 'US Department of Health and Human Services: Public Health Service', that help in understanding some of the terms involved in defining epidemiology.

- *Study:* Epidemiology is a scientific discipline, sometimes called 'the basic science of public health'. It has, at its foundation, sound methods of scientific inquiry.
- *Distribution:* Epidemiology is concerned with the frequency and pattern of health events in a population. Frequency includes not only the number of such events in a population, but also the rate or risk of disease in the population. The rate (number of events divided by size of the population) is critical to epidemiologists because it allows valid comparisons across different populations.
- *Pattern:* It refers to the occurrence of health-related events by time, place, and personal characteristics.

1. Time characteristics include annual occurrence, seasonal occurrence, and daily or even hourly occurrence during an epidemic.
2. Place characteristics include geographic variation, urban-rural differences, and location of worksites or schools.
3. Personal characteristics include demographic factors such as age, race, sex, marital status, and socio-economic status, as well as behaviours and environmental exposures.

This characterization of the distribution of health-related states or events is one broad aspect of epidemiology called descriptive epidemiology. Descriptive epidemiology provides the *what, who, when,* and *where* of health-related events.

- *Determinants:* Epidemiology is also used to search for causes and other factors that influence the occurrence of health-related events. Analytic epidemiology attempts to provide the *why* and *how* of such events by comparing groups with different rates of disease occurrence and with differences in demographic characteristics, genetic, or immunologic make-up, behaviours, environmental exposures, and other so-called potential risk factors. Under ideal circumstances, epidemiologic findings provide sufficient evidence to direct swift and effective public health control and prevention measures.

- *Health-related states or events:* Originally, epidemiology was concerned with epidemics of communicable diseases. Then epidemiology was extended to endemic communicable diseases and non-communicable infectious diseases. More recently, epidemiologic methods have been applied to chronic diseases, injuries, birth defects, maternal-child health, occupational health, and environmental health. Now, even behaviours related to health and well-being (amount of exercise, seat belt use, etc.) are recognized as valid subjects for applying epidemiologic methods. In these lessons, we use the term 'disease' to refer to the range of health-related states or events.
- *Specified populations:* Although epidemiologists and physicians in clinical practice are both concerned with disease and the control of disease, they differ greatly in how they view 'the patient'. Clinicians are concerned with the health of an individual; epidemiologists are concerned with the collective health of the people in a community or other area. When faced with a patient with diarrhoeal disease, for example, the clinician and the epidemiologist have different responsibilities. Although both are interested in establishing the correct diagnosis, the clinician usually focuses on treating and caring for the individual. The epidemiologist focuses on the exposure (action or source that caused the illness), the number of other persons who may have been similarly exposed, the potential for further spread in the community, and interventions to prevent additional cases or recurrences.
- *Application:* Epidemiology is more than 'the study of'. As a discipline within public health, epidemiology provides data for directing public health action. However, using epidemiologic data is an art as well as a science. To treat a patient, a clinician must call upon experience and creativity as well as scientific knowledge. Similarly, an epidemiologist not only uses the

scientific methods of descriptive and analytic epidemiology in 'diagnosing' the health of a community, but also must call upon experience and creativity when planning how to control and prevent disease in the community.

Although epidemiologic thinking has been traced from Hippocrates (circa 400 BC) through Graunt (1662), Farr and Snow (both mid-1800s), and others, the discipline did not blossom until the end of the Second World War. The contributions of some of these early and more recent thinkers are described as follows.

Hippocrates (about 400 BC) attempted to explain disease occurrence from a rational instead of a supernatural viewpoint. In his essay entitled 'On airs, waters and places', Hippocrates suggested that environmental and host factors such as behaviours might influence the development of disease (McKenzie, Pinger, and Kotecki, 2005). However, it was not until the nineteenth century that the distribution of disease in specific human population groups was measured to any large extent. This work marked not only the formal beginnings of epidemiology, but also some of its most spectacular achievements.

Another early contributor to epidemiology was John Graunt, the London haberdasher, who published his landmark analysis of mortality data in 1662. He was the first to quantify patterns of birth, death, and disease occurrence, noting male-female disparities, high infant mortality, urban-rural differences, and seasonal variations. No one built upon Graunt's work until the mid-1800s, when William Farr began to systematically collect and analyse Britain's mortality statistics. Farr, considered the father of modern vital statistics and surveillance, developed many of the basic practices used today in vital statistics and disease classification. He extended the epidemiologic analysis of morbidity and mortality data, looking at the effects of marital status, occupation, and altitude. He also developed many epidemiologic concepts and techniques which are still in use today.

Meanwhile, an anaesthesiologist named John Snow was conducting a series of investigations in London that later earned him the title 'the father of field epidemiology'. The finding by John Snow (1954) that the risk of cholera in London was related to the drinking of water supplied by a particular company provides a well-known account of epidemiological work (Aggleton, 1990; Bonita, Beaglehole and Kjellström, 2006).

Milton Terris, a leading exponent of close interrelationships among epidemiology, public health, and policy, has summarized the functions of epidemiology as:

1. Discover the agent, host, and environmental factors that affect health, in order to provide the scientific basis for the prevention of disease and injury and the promotion of health.
2. Determine the relative importance of causes of illness, disability, and death, in order to establish priorities for research and action.
3. Identify those sections of the population that have the greatest risk from specific causes of ill health (and benefit from specific interventions), in order that the indicated action may be directed appropriately.
4. Evaluate the effectiveness of preventive and therapeutic health programmes and services in improving the health of the population.
5. Study the natural history of disease from its precursor states through its manifestations and clinical course.
6. Conduct surveillance of disease and injury occurrence in populations and of the levels of risk factors—passive (receive reports) and active (poll practitioners, conduct surveys).
7. Investigate outbreaks (e.g., hospital-acquired infections, disease clusters, food-borne and water-borne infections) to identify their source and controlling epidemics (e.g., measles, rubella, coronary heart disease, overweight).

'The epidemiological approach to lifestyle derives from a multicausal model of disease that includes social and environmental factors and it is primarily concerned with identifying risk factors for disease. These are identified through the collection of population health and demographic data and statistical analysis. However, the focus of epidemiological research is prediction rather than understanding' (Hansen and Easthop, 2007: 35). Sociologists and some medical anthropologists have queried the basis of many of the epidemiological claims about lifestyle and disease, and argued that epidemiological understandings of lifestyle are not effective ways of explaining patterns of health and illness. Cockerham (1995: 90) defines health lifestyles as 'patterns of voluntary behaviour based on choices from options that are available according to their (individual's) life situations'. Abel (1991: 900) describes health lifestyles as 'patterns of health related behaviour, values and attitudes adapted by groups of individuals in response to their social, cultural and economic situation. Thus, from sociological perspective, lifestyle factors and lifestyles are constrained by material resources in addition to cultural and symbolic values. Sociological arguments about social location and health focus on how life chances shaped by an individual's social location impact on their health, for example, through social opportunities, material advantage/disadvantage, living conditions, working conditions, and access to education and social support.'

Hansen and Easthop (2007), citing from different sources write: 'In many epidemiological studies about the causes of common diseases such as heart disease, class is excluded from the statistical analysis because it (inequality and socio-economic status) has the largest causative impact on patterns of disease.' However, according to White (2002), when epidemiologists focus on the proximate causes of disease, diet, cholesterol, and hypertension, for example, they individualize the causes of disease and miss the distant social causes. As Link and Phelan (1995) argue, we need to contextualize risk factors so as to see how individuals are exposed to them and have limited access to resources to respond to them. It is the lack of resources to respond to risks that is the fundamental cause of disease patterns. If we want to change the patterns of disease, then we must change the distant, not the proximate causes. 'Sociological position on lifestyle is frequently attributed to Weber who considered that while choice is 'the major factor in the operationalization of a lifestyle', 'the actualization of choices is influenced by life chances'. Life chances are the chances that people have because of their position in life. This includes factors such as gender, age, education, employment, income, and property as well as rights, norms, and social relationships. 'Hence, lifestyles are not random behaviours unrelated to structure but are typically deliberate choices influenced by life chances" (Cockerham et al., 1997: 325). In addition, when discussing the social, cultural, and economic situation within which patterns of health are formed, sociological writers have emphasized that the social causes of ill health are closely related to social inequalities (Navarro, 1976). In fact, inequality is viewed by many sociologists as the most important social factor impacting on health and disease (Wilkinson, 2005). The outcome of the unequal distribution of political, economic, and social resources necessary for a healthy life is the social gradient of health (White, 2002). As evidence, sociologists point to the differential health outcomes of different social groups such as men and women, indigenous and non-indigenous, rural/urban dwellers, the unemployed, and students (Hansen and Easthop, 2007).

Epidemiology essentially deals with rates of disease and mortality and has always acknowledged multiple and interactive causes of ill health. Epidemiology has always been one of the basic sciences in preventive and clinical medicine. Its first major impact was on the understanding of the aetiology and the natural history of infectious diseases and on the design and implementation of effective control measures for these diseases. With the reduction in infectious diseases in the twentieth century, increasing epidemiological attention was focused on identifying the determinants of chronic diseases associated with an ageing population and modern living conditions, such as osteoporosis, cataracts, stroke, diabetes, cancer, heart disease, and arthritis. These diseases almost certainly have multiple determinants such as diet, genetic, psychosocial, and occupational factors, and level of physical activity (and in some cases infectious factors).

Epidemiologists are concerned not only with death, illness (people who are sick), and disability, but also with more positive health states and most importantly with the means to improve health. 'Epidemiologists are usually interested in at least three things. The first is the distribution of disease within a particular group or population. Here they may wish to find out who is most affected, what their characteristics are, and where they are located. Their second interest is in the causes of disease. By examining disease patterns, it is often possible to identify its causes. For example, John Snow's study of the 1854 cholera epidemic in London led him to notice that the disease was particularly prevalent in the area surrounding a particular water pump—the broad street water pump in Soho. This led him to suggest that the disease in societies might be spread by contaminated water: a view that has since proved to be correct but at that time it ran contrary to most medical opinion. Finally, epidemiologists may be interested in what happens after someone has a disease. Here, they may find themselves plotting the course taken by particular diseases, the effectiveness of different kinds of therapies, and the likely outcome if treatment does not take place' (Aggleton, 1990: 19).

Aggleton further says that 'in carrying out their work, epidemiologists measure health in a variety of ways. Two of these measures are of particular importance. First, they may be interested in mortality—the ages at which people die and the causes of death. Second, they may be interested in morbidity or sickness' (1990: 19)

The study of mortality is an important area of social epidemiology, particularly in societies that are less developed and are affected more by acute conditions than chronic conditions. Mortality refers to the death process characterizing a population. The study of mortality examines the relationship between death and the size, composition, and distribution of the population. Furthermore, they are also engaged in investigating the 'who, how, why, and when' issues related to dying, and expectation of life, infant mortality, etc.

According to Thomas (2002), mortality like fertility is significantly influenced by socio-cultural factors, and even age-specific deaths are to a certain extent a function of non-biological factors. These include characteristics such as marital status and family structure, socio-economic status, occupation, industry and employment status, lifestyle, and even religion.

The study of morbidity is perhaps the most important dimension of social epidemiology, particularly in modern industrialized societies. Morbidity or the level of sickness and disability within a population, historically, has been an area of study for both clinicians and population-oriented scientists such as epidemiologists. In recent years, however, increased activity on the part of social scientists has been observed, as researchers apply various methodologies and perspectives to the study of sickness and disability. The health status of a population is reflected in the levels of morbidity and the treatment seeking behaviours of its members.

Morbidity or sickness can be measured in a variety of ways. Some of these measures focus on disease, whereas others are more concerned with illness. This can create problems when comparisons are made between different sets of statistics. When examining morbidity statistics, it is important to be clear which of these two dimensions of health they focus on.

The discipline of epidemiology involves the study of the prevalence and incidence of disease and illness. Valuable statistical data about morbidity can be obtained from hospital records, consultations between patients and doctors, records detailing the causes of absence from work, and special surveys. Regardless of the kinds of data collected, epidemiologists take care to distinguish between the incidence of a disease or illness and its prevalence. 'By the term incidence or incidence rate, they mean the number of new cases of a disease or condition occurring over a certain time period expressed as a number per 1,000, 10,000, or 1,00,000 populations at risk' (Coe, 1970: 36). By the term prevalence or prevalence rate, they mean the number of people who actually have the disease or illness at a particular moment. Knowing these numbers, plus the total number at risk, it is possible to calculate the incidence rate and the prevalence rate (usually per 10,000 or per 1,00,000 populations) for a specific disease or illness.

'The incidence rate is one of the valuable measures in epidemiological investigations. If a new or mysterious condition afflicts a population, epidemiologists can trace the spread of the condition through the population by backtracking using incidence data. The cause or origin of a new disease can often only be determined by identifying the characteristics of the victims and the conditions under which the disease was contracted. The exact date of occurrence becomes crucial if the epidemiological detective is to link the onset to a particular set of circumstances. Quite often the key is the socio-cultural characteristics of the victims' (Thomas, 2002: 168). The prevalence rate includes the total number of persons with AIDS divided by the population at risk. In this instance, the population at risk is the total population, since this is a prevalence rate and the entire population is theoretically at risk.

Data on prevalence and incidence become much more useful if these are converted into rates. According to Bonita, Beaglehole, and Kjellström (2006: 18), 'A rate is calculated by dividing the number of cases by the corresponding number of people in the population at risk and is expressed as cases per 10^n people. Some epidemiologists use the term 'rate' only for measurements of disease occurrence per time unit (week, year, etc.)'.

Prevalence: Prevalence (P) of a disease is calculated as follows:

$$\text{Prevalence} = \frac{\textit{Number of people with the disease or condition at a specified time}}{\textit{Number of people in the population at risk at the specified time}} (\times 10^n)$$

Data on the population at risk are not always available and in many studies the total population in the study area is used as an approximation.

Bonita, Beaglehole, and Kjellström (2006) further add, 'prevalence is often expressed as cases per 100 (percentage) or per 1,000 population. In this case, P has to be multiplied by the appropriate factor: 10^n. If the data have been collected for one point in time, P is the 'point prevalence rate'. It is sometimes more convenient to use the 'period prevalence rate', calculated as the total number of cases at any time during a specified period, divided by the population at risk midway through the period. Similarly, 'lifetime prevalence' is the total number of persons known to have had the disease for at least some part of their lives' (Bonita, Beaglehole, and Kjellström, 2006: 19).

Incidence refers to the rate at which new events occur in a population. Incidence takes into account the variable time periods during which individuals are disease-free and thus 'at risk' of developing the disease. In the calculation of incidence, the numerator is the number of new events that occur in a defined time period, and the denominator is the population at risk of experiencing the event during this period. The most accurate way of calculating incidence is to calculate what last calls the 'person-time incidence rate'. Each person in the study population contributes one person-year to the denominator for each year (or day, week, month) of observation before disease develops, or the person is lost to follow-up.

Incidence (I) is calculated as follows:

$$\text{Incidence} = \frac{\textit{Number of new events in a specified period}}{\textit{Number of persons exposed to risk during this period}} (\times 10^n)$$

The numerator strictly refers only to first events of disease. The units of incidence rate must always include a unit of time (cases per 10^n and per day, week, month, year, etc.) (Bonita, Beaglehole, and Kjellström).

Social Epidemiology

According to Thomas (2002: 157), 'social epidemiology is the branch of epidemiology that deals with the social distribution of disease and the social determinants of health and illness. The field incorporates the concepts and methods of sociology, psychology, political science, economics, demography, geography, and biology. Social epidemiologists examine the origin and spread of various health conditions and the ways in which health is tied to different social factors. Social epidemiology has its roots in medical epidemiology. As the term implies, the medical specialty 'epidemiology' was originally devoted to the study of communicable diseases with epidemic potential. The 'social' dimension was added in the twentieth century and social epidemiology now, more appropriately, applies to virtually any health problem that affects a population. The expanded perspective offered by social epidemiology owes its existence in no small part to the work of medical sociologists during the last half of the twentieth century.'

Social epidemiology is the study of the causes and distribution of health, disease, and impairment throughout a population. 'A key challenge for epidemiology is to sustain a sense of coherence in light of increasing specialization; indeed, in recent decades, myriad branches of the discipline have developed, including pharmacoepidemiology, social epidemiology, genetic epidemiology, and molecular epidemiology. A successful integration of these sub-disciplines and awareness that, increasingly, health issues are global issues may signal a new paradigm, which Mervyn Susser and Ezra Susser have labelled 'eco-epidemiology'. This era would be characterized by a multilevel approach to the study of disease, wherein advances at the molecular, individual, and societal levels of study would be integrated' (Hang, 2008: 615).

Social epidemiologists argue that people are not created equal. 'On the contrary, socio-economic, political, and other processes and structures determine the different and unequal distribution of resources and services that promote health, buffer against illness, and cure disease. Throughout the world, the highest socio-economic classes have the highest-quality shelter, health care, and schools, whereas the lowest classes often struggle with reduced access to affordable food, adequate housing health care, and protection from environmental hazards. Further, it has been argued by the modern social epidemiologists that throughout the history, social elites have inequitably organized societies through laws, policies, and cultural norms in order to protect or benefit their position. As a result, persisting inequalities based on gender class, age, sexual orientation, race and ethnicity, and other characteristics are the rule rather than exception' (Miller, Waning, Bread, and Knapp, 2002: 17–18).

This chapter can be concluded by quoting Hansen and Easthop (2007: 41), 'social epidemiology is a vibrant multidisciplinary field, as is evidenced by the frequent publications by social epidemiologists in sociological, epidemiological, and mainstream medical journals. Social epidemiologists continue to trial new methods of investigating the interconnections between social dimensions such as education, occupation, income, housing, ethnicity, gender, and age and health. They also make use of multidimensional conceptions of health and draw on qualitative research to enrich their statistical analyses. However, despite the apparent explanatory power of social epidemiology, simpler lifestyle/risk factor epidemiology continues to be the more commonly used source of epidemiological knowledge about lifestyle in medical fields and provides the legitimation for many health promotion programmes'.

References

Abel, T. (1991). 'Measuring Health Lifestyles in Comparative Analysis: Theoretical Issues and Empirical Findings', *Social Science and Medicine,* 32(8): 899–908.

Aggleton, P. (1990). *Health*, London: Routledge Publications.

Bonita, R., Beaglehole, R. and Kjellström, T. (2006). *Basic Epidemiology*, second edition, Geneva: World Health Organization.

Coe, R.M. (1970). *Sociology of Medicine*, New York/London: McGraw-Hill Book Company.

Cockerham, W.C. (1995). *Medical Sociology*, 6th edn, Englewood Cliffs, NJ: Prentice Hall.

Cockerham, W.C., Rütten, A. and Abel, T. (1997). 'Conceptualising contemporary health lifestyles: moving beyond Weber', *The Sociological Quarterly*, 38(2): 321–42.

Epidemiology Program Office. (n.d.). *Principles of Epidemiology: An Introduction to Applied Epidemiology and Biostatistics*, second edition, Atlanta, GA: US Department of Health and Human services, Public Health Service, Centres for Disease Control and Prevention, Epidemiology Program Office.

Hang, Y. (2008). *Encyclopaedia of Global Health*, London/New Delhi: Sage Publications.

Hansen, E. and Easthop, G. (2007). *Lifestyle in Medicine*, London/New York: Routledge Taylor and Francis Group.

Link, B.G. and Phelan, J. (1995). 'Social Conditions as Fundamental Causes of Disease', *Journal of Health and Social Behaviour*, 35 (extra issue): 80–94.

McKenzie, J.F., Pinger, R.R. And Kotecki, J.E. (2005). *An Introduction to Community Health*, London: Jones and Bartlett Publishers.

Miller, C., Waning, B., Bread, J. and Knapp, A. (2002). *Social Epidemiology*, Chapter 2, London: Jones and Bartlett Publishers.

Navarro, V. (1976). *Medicine under Capitalism*, New York: Prodist.

Thomas, R.K. (2002). *Society and Health: Sociology for Health Professionals*, New York: Kluwer Academic Publishers.

Turner, B. (2006). *The Cambridge Dictionary of Sociology*, Cambridge: Cambridge University Press.

White, K. (2002). *An Introduction to the Sociology of Health and Illness*, London: Sage Publications.

Wilkinson, R.G. (2005). *The Impact of Inequality: How to Make Sick Societies Healthier*, New York: The New Press.

CHAPTER FIVE

Illness and Sickness

Illness

The study of health, illness, and society covers a wide and diverse range of topics. These include the analysis of medical knowledge; perceptions on and the experiences of health and illness; social and cultural aspects of body; the interactions between patients and health professionals; the patterned nature of health and illness in relation to a wider social structure; the causation of disease; study of people's interpretations of their bodily experiences; food, water, and other bodily requirements; concerns related to the social aspects of the regulation of bodies; and the social organization of both informal and formal health care (Nettleton, 1995). Sociologists, anthropologists, and historians have described the social basis of health and illness in a wide range of studies, including ethnographies of specific communities. They have explored issues of health care, performance of 'the sick role', the construction of mental illness as a disease, the wider creation of medical belief systems, and the relationship between these and the exercise of power and social control.

'By illness we mean a subjective phenomenon, pertaining to an individual's psychological awareness of having a disease, symptoms, or pain and typically modifying his or her social behaviour as a result or in which individuals perceive themselves as not feeling well and therefore may tend to modify their normal behaviour' (Cockerham and Ritchey, 1997: 71). This definition contrasts with that of a disease, which is a physiological dysfunction within an individual. Contrasted with disease, which is a concept of biology—more specifically of pathology, illness is a phenomenon that is apparent to the individual in terms of an altered state of his perception of himself. He feels sick and hence may act in ways that are different from those which might normally be expected of him. Illness is defined as the ill health in which the person identifies themselves with, often based on self-reported mental or physical symptoms (Wikman, Marklund, and Alexanderson, 2005).

According to Nettleton (1995), illness reminds us that the 'normal' functioning of our minds and bodies is central to social interaction. In this respect, the study of illness throws light on the nature of the interaction between the body, the individual, and the society. That is if we cannot rely on our bodies to function 'normally', then our interaction with the social world becomes perilous; our dependency on others may become exacerbated and in turn our sense of self may be challenged. Therefore, it is clear that biophysical changes have significant social consequences. It has been noted earlier from the literature that responses to illness are not simply determined by either the nature of biophysical symptoms or individual motivations, but rather are shaped and imbued by the social, cultural, and ideological context of a person's biography. Thus, illness is at once both a very personal and a very public or social phenomenon.

In order to highlight the social basis of illness some authors distinguish between disease and illness. Kleinman (1988) suggests that disease is a biophysical event and the prime concern of medical practitioners, whereas 'illness refers to how the sick person and members of the family or wider social network perceive, live with and respond to symptoms and disability'. The basic distinction between disease and illness is that by 'disease' we mean an objective phenomenon characterized by altered functioning of a body as a biological organism. However apparent their manifestations, diseases are hidden processes which can only be understood as their observable signs are related to a body of knowledge about the way in which the human organism works. 'By illness, we mean a subjective phenomenon in which individuals perceive themselves as not feeling well and therefore may tend to modify their normal behaviour' (Cockerham and Ritchey, 1997: 71). 'It has been argued by some sociologists that the state of illness is fundamentally different from that of disease. Illness refers to the social, lived experience of symptoms and suffering which is innately human. It includes recognizing that bodily processes are malfunctioning and taking steps to rectify the situation, such as seeking treatment. Disease, on the other hand, is not limited to humans; animals or plants can be diseased. Indeed, to describe someone as 'diseased' implies a lack of humanity. In contrast to illness, the term 'disease' is defined as denoting a technical malfunction or deviation from the biological norm, which is 'scientifically' diagnosed. This definition, of course, does not necessarily imply that disease is an objective state, for, as scholars from the social constructionist perspective argue, the categorizing of disease is influenced by the social, historical, and political context as is the definition of illness' (Lupton, 2003: 93–94).

'Dingwall also argues that there is no such thing as 'essential illness' rather illness is construed through the meanings and interpretations that are accorded to certain categories of experience and 'there is no necessary relationship to any biological happening'. Advocating the need for a phenomenological approach, Dingwall states that Illness action is the outcome of continuing efforts on the part of a sick person, and those with whom he {sick} associates, to make sense of what is going on in the light of knowledge, resources and motivations available to them' (Nettleton,1995: 78, 79).

Thus, rather than simply observing illness behaviour, sociologists must endeavour to understand illness action (Nettleton, 1995). The former refers to the way people behave, given the presence of symptoms, whereas the latter focuses on how people make sense of and interpret their experience regarding their illness and, crucially, what it means to them. When people have spoken about their experience of illness, it becomes evident that these are woven into their biographies. The experience of illness reflects the person's experience of life. Nettleton cites Kleinman's 'illness narrative':

> a story the patient tells, and significant others retell, to give coherence to the distinctive events and long-term course of sufferings. The plot lines, core metaphors, and rhetorical devices that structure the illness narrative are drawn from cultural and personal models for arranging experiences in meaningful ways and for effectively communicating those meanings ... The personal narrative does not merely reflect illness experience, but rather contributes to the experience of symptoms and suffering. (Nettleton, 1995: 78–79)

Given that the interpretation of illness contributes to how it is experienced, Kleinman argues that it is crucial that practitioners understand and take heed of the lay person's story. Williams coined the term 'narrative reconstruction', that is, the routine way in which we make the sense of events in our lives. How people make sense of their illness is within the context of their personal biographies and in turn this must invariably be influenced by, and meshed with, the cultural values of the society in which they live. Sociologists have, therefore, produced descriptions of the everyday situations of particular chronic diseases, and in so doing have highlighted the biographical and cultural context in which illness emerges.

On the one hand, illness is a personal event to the extent that each of us attempts first to evaluate for ourselves the meaning of any symptoms of which we become aware. The point is that as long as what we feel is not communicated to others or what we do is not observed by others, illness remains a personal event. On the other hand, illness becomes a public or social phenomenon when it becomes visible to others and when this leads to modification of the social interaction patterns between the sick man and those around him (Coe, 1970). The awareness by others that a person is ill usually occurs through two routes. First, it may be the result of their observation of the sick person's actions. He may fail to fulfil his normal role expectations or perform them inadequately. The result of person's failure to fulfil his normal role expectations may help people, who are in contact with him, to realize his abnormal behaviour, for example, limping, breathing rapidly, trembling, or exhibiting altered external characteristics (is pale, flushed, etc.). Second, their observation would be supplemented by the sick man communicating his feelings to others. The important thing here is that in different social situations, the opportunity to observe and be told about a person's sickness may vary considerably. The more prolonged and intimate the social contact, the greater the chances for observation of and the communication about the illness. In general, this means that members of one's family and primary groups have a better chance to become aware of illness than do others.

The sociology of health and illness is informed by five theoretical traditions:

1. *Parsonsian functionalism* looks at the role the sick person plays in society. The focus is on how being ill is given a specific form in human societies so that the social system's stability and cohesion can be maintained.
2. *Symbolic interactionism* is concerned with examining the interaction between the different role players in the health and illness drama. The focus is on how illness and the subjective experience of being sick are constructed through the doctor-patient exchange. The argument here is that illness is a social accomplishment among actors rather than just a matter of physiological malfunction.
3. *Marxist theory* is concerned with the relationship between health and illness and capitalist social organization. The main focus is on how the definition and treatment of health and illness are influenced by the nature of economic activity in a capitalist society.
4. *Feminist theory* explores the gendered nature of the definition of illness and treatment of patients. Its main concern is the way in which medical treatment involves men's control over women's bodies and identities.
5. *Foucauldian theory* concentrates on the dominant medical discourse, which has constructed definitions of normality (health) and deviance (sickness). This discourse provides subjects in modern societies with the vocabulary through which their medical needs and remedies are defined. The source and beneficiary of this discourse is the medical profession. Foucauldian theorists also argue that medical

discourse plays an important role in the management of individual bodies (what Foucault called 'anatomo-politics') and bodies *en masse* (bio-politics). Medicine is not just about medicine as it is conventionally understood, but also about wider structures of power and control (for details, please see (www.palgrave.com/bilton/pdfs/0333_945719_14_cha13.pdf).

Chronic and Acute Illness

According to Larkin (2011), several key theoretical insights into the experience of illness as a social state have been developed. These have focused on both acute and chronic illness. The nature of illnesses can be either acute or chronic. Acute illnesses are those which are short-term and curable, such as colds and sickness bugs. Recovery occurs within a few days, with or without medical intervention. Functionalism has been chosen as an example of a theoretical perspective which has provided insights into the experience of acute illness as a social state. The most well-known work on acute illness within this perspective is that of Parsons. He developed the concept of the 'sick role' which he used to explain how the experience of having an acute illness is socially, and not primarily biologically or physiologically, defined.

'Chronic illness refers to those forms of long-term and non-communicable health disorders that interfere with social interaction and role performance. They are also emergent in nature and the stages in their progress can be unpredictable. They usually have an 'insidious onset', and although symptoms may fluctuate and treatments are available, there are no known medical cures or chances of returning to a pre-morbid state. These types of illness require continuous medical intervention and often interfere with social interaction, the ability to carry out everyday roles and the capacity to fulfil social obligations' (Larkin, 2011: 104–105). Larkin further says, chronic illnesses, such as cardiovascular diseases, certain types of cancer, asthma, multiple sclerosis, diabetes, Parkinson's, hypertension, rheumatoid arthritis, migraine, epilepsy, psoriasis, and senile dementia are by definition long-term illnesses. Thus, the impact on sufferers' daily lives, their social relationships, their identity (the view that others hold of them), their sense of self (their private view of themselves), and those around them is inevitably more profound. Furthermore, people can simultaneously suffer from two or more chronic illnesses. This is referred to as co-morbidity and examples of co-morbid chronic conditions are diabetes, Alzheimer's, asthma, and cardiovascular disease. Several 'new' chronic illnesses have also been relatively recently identified. Among these are HIV/AIDS, stress, anorexia nervosa, bulimia, and obesity.

Illness and Sickness

In a basic sense, a state of illness or sickness constitutes 'ill health' and is the converse of a state of 'health'. However, the subjective nature of conditions of health and illness has led medical sociologists to formulate a more complicated depiction of these concepts. A major distinction in this regard is made between illness and sickness. According to Thomas (2002), illness refers to the individual, private, and usually biological aspect of the state of ill health. The term 'illness' relates to the set of symptoms known only to the individual and in this sense is private as opposed to public. It is argued that illness (but not sickness) is a state shared by human beings with all other animals; that is, it is a state of biological dysfunction known only to the individual organism. Under this definition, it could be contended that the actual level of illness is similar from society to society, reflecting the primarily biological nature of illness.

'Sickness refers to the public or social component of ill health. Illness is transformed into sickness when the condition becomes publicly known through announcement by the affected party, observation by significant others, or professional diagnosis. Thus, while illness is primarily a biological state, sickness is a social state. Sickness is social not only because it is recognized beyond the bounds of the individual *per se*, but also because it has implications for social role performance and interpersonal interaction' (Thomas, 2002: 23).

Thomas further says, 'some simple examples may help clarify the distinction between illness and sickness. An individual who feels bad (e.g., headache and nausea) is clearly ill. However, if the individual never discloses his or her symptoms to others (or they go unobserved by others) and continues to perform social roles adequately, he or she, although 'ill', would not be considered 'sick'. Conversely, if an individual is unable to perform social roles due to some generalized condition, although clinically identifiable symptoms cannot be found, this individual would be considered 'sick'. Unlike illness, the amount of sickness varies widely from society to society and within the same society at different time periods. The amount of sickness reflects the perceptions of society at that point in time. This means that the level of sickness is much more 'elastic' than the level of illness. Examples of the elasticity of sickness can be found during wartime when military physicians at induction centres adopt a quite different standard of what constitutes disability than in peacetime' (Thomas, 2002: 23–24).

Illness Behaviour

Illness behaviour is an important variable in medical sociology because not everyone responds the same way when sick. Some people go to physicians for treatment when they experience symptoms of illness, while others with the same symptoms may attempt self-care or dismiss the symptoms as not needing attention. Some people may even deny the experience of symptoms out of anxiety for what the symptoms may mean (e.g., AIDS, cancer). Subjective interpretations of feeling states when ill are the basis of illness behaviour. Models of illness behaviour have been developed by Parsons in his well-known concept of the sick role.

According to Mechanic (1986), illness behaviour arises in response to circumstances that challenge the ongoing homeostasis. People are extraordinarily adaptive, but some changes in the situation, whether arising within the organism or from external factors, induce self-consciousness and appraisal, and require assessments about the nature of the problem, its causes, and the strategies to be initiated. These responses are both cognitive and affective, concerned with understanding the changes and maintaining emotional equilibrium. Illness behaviour is more than a psychological response among persons faced with a situation calling for assessment. It also arises in response to troubling social situations and may serve as an effective means of achieving release from social expectations, as an excuse for failure, or as a way of obtaining a variety of privileges including monetary compensation.

Moreover, the physician and other health personnel may be an important source of social support and may be particularly important for patients lacking strong social ties.

'Mechanic and Volkart identified four dimensions of the illness that influenced the decision to seek medical help: (1) the frequency with which the illness occurs in a given population (its commonality); (2) the familiarity of the symptoms; (3) the predictability of the outcome of the illness; and (4) the amount of threat and loss that is likely to result from the illness. In later studies, Mechanic (1978) identified a number of other factors relating to the type of illness that influenced help-seeking behaviour. These included the visibility of the symptoms, the perceived present and future seriousness of the symptoms, the extent to which symptoms disrupt social activities, the frequency of symptoms and interpretations of the cause of symptoms, and availability of treatment. In addition, Mechanic recognized that the impact that illness had on those caring for the patient was an important determinant of illness behaviour. He suggested that when illness becomes so disruptive to everyday life that the carer is unable to cope any longer, medical help will usually be sought' (Gabe, Bury, and Elson, 2004: 65–66).

According to Gabe, Bury, and Elson (2004), 'Zola identified five factors, or 'triggers', which initiate a person to consulting the doctor. First, there is the occurrence of an interpersonal crisis, such as the death of relative. Although the patient may experience symptoms for some time, it often takes a crisis to occur before they seek medical help. Second is perceived interference with social or personal relations, where symptoms start to have an impact on a person's social life or their relationships with others. The third trigger is sanctioning, where family members or friends suggest that they seek medical help and thereby agree that there is a need to go to the doctor. Fourth is perceived interference with vocational or physical activity, where symptoms prevent the patient from carrying out their daily activities. Finally, there is the temporalizing of symptoms, where a time limit is placed on the illness. People will often say that they will consult the doctor if the symptom has not gone within a given time frame.' Although the decision to consult the doctor is shaped by the type of illness and a person's individual and social circumstances, it is unusual for a person to seek medical help without first discussing their symptoms with at least one other person. A number of studies have shown that most people talk with many different friends and family members before going to see a doctor. This line of communication about illness has been termed 'the lay referral system' and has been shown to influence illness behaviour' (2004: 65–67).

Gabe, Bury, and Elson (2004) also cite Herzlich (1973) who described three ways in which people viewed their illness: (1) illness as destructive; (2) illness as a liberator; and (3) illness as an occupation. 'Where illness was perceived as destructive, it was seen as a barrier to maintaining normal roles within society, which eventually resulted in exclusion from social groups. People perceiving illness in this way often used denial as a means of restricting social isolation and they therefore tended not to consult the doctor. Those who considered illness as a liberator viewed it as a positive experience where they were freed from their social obligations. Medical advice was generally sought as it provided legitimate entrance to the sick role. Where illness was seen as an occupation, it was considered as something that had to be worked at in much the same way as was required of paid employment or domestic work. The maximum medical advice was therefore sought in order to fight the illness' (Gabe, Bury, and Elson, 2004: 66).

Mental Illness

'Mental health is the state of successful performance of mental function, resulting in productive activities, fulfilling relationships with other people, and the ability to adapt to change and to cope with adversity' (McKenzie, Pinger, and Kotecki, 2005: 307). WHO (1981) defines mental health as 'the capacity of the individual, the group and the environment to interact with one another in ways that promote subjective well-being, the optimal development and use of mental abilities (cognitive, affective and relational), the achievement of individual and collective goals consistent with justice, and the attainment and preservation of conditions of fundamental equality' (Gangolli, Duggal, and Shukla, 2005: 127).

According to McKenzie, Pinger, and Kotecki (2005: 308), 'mental illness is a term that refers collectively to all diagnosable mental disorders. Mental disorders are health conditions that are characterized by alterations in thinking, mood, or behaviour (or some combination thereof) associated with distress and/or impaired functioning. People with mental illness have organic or metabolic (biochemical) disorders that prevent them from functioning effectively and happily in society. Many people with mental illness can be treated successfully with medications and are thus able to live successfully in our communities.'

Thomas (2002) explains various models that can be used in defining mental health and illness. According to Thomas, 'from a medical model perspective, mental health would be thought of as simply the absence of symptoms of mental illness. From this perspective, mental illness refers collectively to all diagnosable mental disorders or health conditions that are characterized by alterations in thinking, mood, or behaviour (or some combination thereof) associated with distress and/or impaired functioning. Proponents of the medical model often view mental disorders as having physiological/anatomical foundations and prescribe physiological/anatomical treatment. While the medical model is not a very comfortable fit with most notions of mental health and illness, this model has continued to exert significant influence due to the role of psychiatrists whose approval is typically required for treatment, hospital admission or discharge, and drug prescription' (2002: 300–301).

Thomas examines the functional model of mental health also. According to this model, 'mental health can be defined as a state of successful mental functioning, resulting in productive activities, fulfilling relationships, and the ability to adapt to change and cope with adversity' (ibid.: 301).

According to the psychological model, 'the individual can make a rational decision as to whether he is sick or well. This assumption does not hold when dealing with individuals with conditions that might cause them to have a distorted notion of their ability to function' (ibid.: 302). According to Thomas, 'a model that relates specifically to mental illness is the societal reaction model. Proponents of this perspective contend that there is no such thing as mental illness in a scientific sense. Mental illness is a concept constructed by society as a means of controlling residual deviant behaviour, i.e., behaviour that does not fit nicely into the sin or crime categories but is nevertheless found to be objectionable. It is no surprise that those who are typically labelled as mentally ill are those who are on the margins of society and relatively powerless. The societal reaction approach argues that certain behaviours of certain categories of people are selectively chosen for labelling as mental illness' (ibid.: 302). Thomas also explains the legal model of mental illness. 'The legal model has more application with regard to mental illness than physical illness. All states have laws that afford the authorities the ability to ascertain the competency of individuals to manage their affairs, stand trial, and otherwise act competently. Although input from the mental health system is required, the standard is ultimately a legal one. Thus, individuals may be legally adjudged too sick to manage their affairs, stand trial, or make decisions with regard to their own treatment' (ibid.: 302). Mary Larkin (2011) also explains different types of mental illnesses and disorders, which range considerably in their degree of seriousness. Anxiety disorders, depression, bipolar disorder, schizophrenia, dementia, personality disorders, anorexia nervosa, and bulimia are some of the examples of such mental illness and disorders. A brief description of these examples as given by Larkin (2011: 122–123) is given below:

- *Anxiety disorders:* People with these disorders experience constant worry and fear that interferes with their normal functioning. There are many different types of anxiety disorder and they include panic disorder, obsessive-compulsive disorder, posttraumatic stress disorder, social anxiety disorder, specific phobias, and generalized anxiety disorder.
- *Depression:* This happens when feelings of sadness, worthlessness, and loneliness are very intense and last for long periods of time. This illness is also referred to as unipolar depression.
- *Bipolar disorder:* This involves elevated mood states (known as 'hypomania') alternating with depression. Nearly 60 per cent of people with bipolar disorder also misuse drugs or alcohol, which makes accurate diagnosis difficult.
- *Schizophrenia:* This has been linked to unusual activity of chemicals (neurotransmitters) in the brain which leads to those parts of the brain responsible for emotion and sensation

not working properly. Thought processes become distorted and, when severe, sufferers experience intense panic, anger, over-activity, hallucinations, and delusions. As a result, schizophrenia may prevent a person from living a normal life and lead to their withdrawal from those around them.

- *Dementia:* This is a syndrome that is associated with ongoing damage to the structure of the brain. Hence, an individual's ability to understand, speak, remember, control their emotions, and behave appropriately in social situations declines. Aspects of personality may also change.
- *Personality disorders:* These result in recurrent and enduring disturbances in conduct (such as being abnormally rigid and maladaptive) and are associated with dysfunctional interpersonal relationships. There are many different types of personality disorder, for example, paranoid, schizoid, obsessive-compulsive, and histrionic.
- *Anorexia nervosa:* This is a condition whereby people develop an obsession about food and their weight. This causes people to think they are fat when they are actually very underweight. Anorexia seriously damages health and can be fatal.
- *Bulimia:* Another eating disorder in which people go on eating binges and then force themselves to vomit the food they have eaten or use diet pills, laxatives, or diuretics to prevent themselves from gaining weight. These binge-and-purge episodes typically occur at least twice a week.

Larkin (2011) concludes, when discussing the incidence of mental illness, it is important to consider the way that it persists across generations. The children of those with a mental illness may also experience mental ill health because untreated mental illness in a parent can affect their children's social and mental development. This in turn leads to emotional problems and educational failure, both of which can adversely affect future employment. These factors increase their own risk of mental illness in their later lives. In addition, mental illness has negative economic consequences through lost employment, and it is now the most expensive health problem of all. Furthermore, the predicted rise in the numbers of those suffering from mental ill health means that mental health service costs are projected to increase by 45 per cent by 2026.

Causes of Mental Illness

In many cultures, both medical and traditional explanations are used to understand the causes of ill health. Traditional models are often related to spiritual or supernatural causes, such as bad spirits or witchcraft. Few causes related to causation of mental illness are as follows:

- *Stressful life events:* Life is full of experiences and events. Some of these may make a person feel worried and under stress. Most people will learn how to deal with such events and carry on with life. However, sometimes they can lead to mental illness. Life events that cause great stress include unemployment, the death of a loved one, and economic problems such as being in debt, loneliness, infertility, marital conflict, violence, and trauma.
- *Difficult family background:* People who have had an unhappy childhood because of violence or emotional neglect are more likely to suffer mental illnesses such as depression and anxiety later in life.
- *Brain diseases:* Mental retardation, dementias, and emotional problems can result from brain infections, AIDS, head injuries, epilepsy, and strokes. No definite brain pathology has yet been identified for many mental illnesses. However, there is evidence to show that many illnesses are associated with changes in brain chemicals such as neurotransmitters.
- *Heredity or genes:* Heredity is an important factor for severe mental disorders. However, if one parent has a mental illness, the risk that the children will suffer from a mental illness is very small. This is because, like diabetes and heart disease, these disorders are also influenced by environmental factors.
- *Medical problems:* Physical illnesses such as kidney and liver failure can sometimes cause a severe mental disorder. Some medicines (e.g., some of those used to treat high blood pressure) can cause a depressive illness. Many medicines when used in large doses in elderly people can cause a delirium (for details, please see www.rcpsych.ac.uk/files/samplechapter/75_7.pdf).

- *Social factors:* Thomas (2002) also talks about some of the social factors responsible for mental health and illness. Some of these are: age, sex, race, marital status, living arrangements, socio-economic status etc.

References

Cockerham, W.C. and Ritchey, F.J. (1997). *Dictionary of Medical Sociology*, London: Greenwood Press.

Coe, R.M. (1970). *Sociology of Medicine*, New York/London: McGraw-Hill Book Company.

Gabe, J., Bury, M. and Elson, M. (2004). *Key Concepts in Medical Sociology*, London: Sage Publications.

Gangolli, L.V., Duggal, R. and Shukla, A. (2005). *Review of Healthcare in India*, Mumbai: Centre for Enquiry into Health and Allied Themes, Research Centre of Anusandhan Trust, Survey No. 2804 and 2805.

Kleinman, A. (1988). *The Illness Narratives: Suffering, Healing and the Human Condition*, New York: Basic Books.

Larkin, M. (2011). *Social Aspects of Health, Illness and Healthcare*, New York: Open University Press.

Lupton, D. (2003). *Medicine as Culture; Illness, Disease and the Body in Western Societies*, second edition, London: Sage Publications.

McKenzie, J.F., Pinger, R.R. And Kotecki, J.E. (2005). *An Introduction to Community Health*, London: Jones and Bartlett Publishers.

Mechanic, D. (1978). *Medical Sociology*, New York: The Free Press.

———. (1986). 'The Concept of Illness Behaviour: Culture, Situation and Personal Predisposition', *Psychological Medicine*, 16.

Nettleton, S. (1995). *The Sociology of Health and Illness*, UK: Polity Press.

Thomas, R.K. (2002). *Society and Health: Sociology for Health Professionals*, New York: Kluwer Academic Publishers.

Wikman, A., Marklund, S. and Alexanderson, K. (2005). 'Illness, Disease, and Sickness Absence: An Empirical Test of Differences Between Concepts of Ill Health', *Journal of Epidemiology and Community Health.*

Chapter Six

Disease

Types, Agents, Cost, and Prevention

Concept of Disease

Literally the term 'disease' means 'lack of ease or comfort', thus underlining the fact that health is characterized by a sense of well-being (Porta, 2008). Disease is a universal phenomenon. From the functionalist view, it can be said that 'disease' is a social fact. It is experienced by all societies, external to individuals and capable of exerting external constraints on the behaviour of individuals. There is no universally accepted definition of 'disease' but there have been many attempts to define disease. Webster's dictionary defines disease as 'a condition in which body health is impaired, a departure from the normal state of health, an alteration of the human body interrupting the performance of vital functions'. Oxford English dictionary defines disease as 'a condition of the body or some part or organ of the body in which its functions are disrupted or deranged'. Disease is a departure from the state of health. However, Cockerham and Ritchey (1997: 34) mention that a 'disease is considered an adverse physical state consisting of a physiological dysfunction within an individual, as compared to an illness (psychological awareness of a disease) or a sickness (a social state)'. From a sociological point of view, disease is considered as a social phenomenon, occurring in all societies and defined and fought in terms of the particular forces prevalent in the society. The simplest definition is, of course, that disease is just the opposite of health—that is, any deviation from normal functioning or state of complete physical, social, and mental well-being—since health and disease are mutually exclusive (Park, 2009).

The WHO has defined health, but not disease. This is because disease has many shades (spectrum of disease) ranging from in apparent (subclinical cases) to serve manifest illness. Some diseases commence acutely (e.g., food poisoning) and some insidiously (e.g., mental illness, rheumatoid arthritis). In some diseases, a carrier state occurs in which the individual remains outwardly healthy and is able to infect others (e.g., typhoid fever). In some instances, the same organism may cause more than one clinical manifestation (streptococcus). In some cases, the same disease may be caused by more than one organism (e.g., diarrhoea). Some disease have a short course, and some a prolonged course. It is easy to determine the illness when the signs and symptoms are manifest, but in many diseases the border line between normal and abnormal is indistinct as in the case of diabetes, hypertension, and mental illness. The end-point of final outcome of disease is variable—recovery, disability, or death of the host.

Biomedical model of disease and illness regards them as the consequence of certain malfunctions of the human body. The biomedical model of disease is based on the following assumptions:

- Disease is an organic condition: non-organic factors associated with the human mind are considered unimportant or are ignored altogether in the search for biological causes of pathological symptoms.
- Disease is a temporary organic state that can be eradicated/cured by medical intervention.
- Disease is experienced by a sick individual, who then becomes the object of treatment.
- Disease is treated after the symptoms appear—the application of medicine is a reactive healing process.
- Disease is treated in a medical environment—a surgery or a hospital—away from the site where the symptoms first appeared.

This model has dominated medical practice because it has been seen to work. It is based on a technically powerful science that has made a massive contribution to key areas of health (e.g., vaccination). However, Anthony Giddens (2006) says that over the past few decades, the biomedical model of disease and health has been the object of growing criticism.

Assumptions and critiques of the biomedical model of disease and illness

	Assumptions	*Critiques*
1.	Disease is the breakdown of the human body caused by a specific biological agent.	Disease is socially constructed, not something that can be revealed through 'scientific truth'.
2.	The patient is passive being whose 'sick body' can be treated separately from his or her mind.	The patient's opinions and experience of illness is crucial to the treatment. The Patient is an active, 'whole' being whose overall well-being—not just physical health—is important.
3.	Medical specialists possess 'expert knowledge' and prescribe the only valid treatment of disease.	Medical experts are not the only source of knowledge about health and illness. Alternative forms of knowledge are equally valid.
4.	The appropriate arena for the treatment is the hospital, where medical technology is concentrated and best employed.	Healing does not need to take place in a hospital. Treatments utilizing technology, mediation, and surgery are not necessarily superior.

Richard K. Thomas (2002) mentions that originally referring to a state of 'disease', the term has come to be used in a variety of ways. The most significant one involves the identification of a medically recognized pathological condition. Technically, this means a syndrome involving clinically identifiable and measurable signs and symptoms reflecting underlying biological pathology. This view of disease clearly reflects an orientation derived from a health care environment dominated by infectious illnesses. This conceptualization continues to be important, since it underlies the medical model perspective on health and illness and is the definition instilled in health professionals. In medical sociology, a disease is considered an adverse physical state consisting of a physiological dysfunction within an individual, as compared to illness or sickness. In actual practice, the term 'disease' is applied rather liberally to a wide variety of conditions that do not precisely fit the definition.

Diagnosis of a disease is made by correlating the observable signs or symptoms of a disease with knowledge about the functioning of the human organism (Coe, 1970). Thus, understanding of disease depends upon observations of altered, abnormal states of the human organism. These signs may be objectively observed and even measurable, such as elevated body temperature or skin rash, or they may be subjective symptoms, such as pain in the back, etc. Many of the signs are not directly observable and it has been one of the basic sources of the success of modern medicine to have found methods for taking 'readings' of bodily function, which allow a skilled observer to pick up signs which he would ordinarily not be able to sense. The stethoscopei—nvented by Laennec in 1816—is a case in point.

Social Causes of Disease and Death

People get sick and die partly due to natural causes. One person may have a genetic predisposition to cancer. Another may come in contact with the deadly Ebola virus in the environment. However, over and above such natural causes of illness and death, Brym and Lie (2007) have singled out some of the social causes also. Some of the important social causes are given here:

1. *Lifestyle factor:* Cigarette smoking, excessive use of alcohol and drugs, poor diet, lack of exercise, and social isolation are associated with poor health and premature death. According to the official statistics, the best available estimates for the United States suggest that the three leading background causes of death in 2000 were tobacco use, poor diet and physical inactivity, and alcohol consumption. A third of the people who smoke are likely to die prematurely from smoking-related illnesses. This amounts to about 4,35,000 Americans annually. About 30 per cent of all cancer deaths in the United States result from tobacco use, and smoking is also a leading cause of heart disease. Many experts believe that poor diet and physical inactivity will soon overtake tobacco as the leading background cause of death. Today, poor diet and physical inactivity are responsible for death of about 4,00,000 Americans every year. They are leading causes of heart disease and are implicated in about 35 per cent of all cancer deaths;

poor diet and physical inactivity is especially a big problem in poor neighbourhoods.

2. *Social situation:* Social isolation too affects one's chance of becoming ill and dying prematurely. Thus, unmarried people have a greater chance of dying prematurely than older people. At any age, the death of a spouse increases one's chance of dying, while remarrying decreases one's chance of dying. Social class, caste, ethnicity, etc., define an individual's social situation. Many a time, social situation may lead to isolation and marginalization. Social isolation is a particularly big problem among elderly people who retire, lose a spouse and friends, and cannot rely on family members or state institutions for social support. Such people are prone to fall into a state of depression that contributes to ill health.
3. *Public health system:* The public health system is composed of government-run programmes that ensure access to clean drinking water, basic sewage and sanitation services, and inoculation against infectious diseases. The absence of a public health system is associated with high rates of illness, disease, and low life expectancy. The health care system is a component of the public health system. It is composed of a nation's clinics, hospitals, and other facilities for ensuring health and treating illness. The absence of a system that ensures access by citizens to a minimum standard of health care is also associated with high rates of disease and low life expectancy. Exposure to all three sets of social causes of illness and death is strongly related to country of residence, class, race, and gender.
4. *Basic health goods:* Nutrition, food, safe drinking water, and sanitation are the basic needs of every human being and the present author categorize them as Basic Health Goods (BHGs). The BHGs have huge bearing on the health condition of the individual and community. Lack of availability, accessibility, and affordability of the BHGs is an important cause of prevalence of disease among various social categories in different parts of the world, including India. A crisis caused by lack of BHGs gradually gets translated into malfunctioning of the human body in several possible forms. There are evidences

that such malfunctioning, over a period of time, take the form of disease. Sometimes, such effects become chronic or even get genetically transmitted. Lack of availability of food, nutrition, potable water, or sanitation is important cause of disease and premature death. However, the social environment (along with the political and economic system) is more responsible for such causation of disease or death than the individual or the community. Government's inability to provide BHGs to its people is dehealthism, a term coined and defined by the present author.

Classification of Diseases

Diseases and health problems can be classified in several meaningful ways. The public often classifies diseases by organ or organ system, such as kidney disease, heart disease, respiratory infection, and so on. Another method of classification is by causative agent—viral disease, chemical poisoning, physical injury, and so forth. In this scheme, causative agents may be biological, chemical, or physical. Biological agents include viruses, rickettsiae, bacteria, protozoa, fungi, and metazoa (multicellular organisms). Chemical agents include drugs, pesticides, industrial chemicals, food additives, air pollutants, and cigarette smoke. Physical agents that can cause injury or disease include various forms of energy such as heat, ultraviolet light, radiation, noise vibrations, and speeding or falling objects. But in community health, diseases are usually classified as acute or chronic, or as communicable (infectious) and non-communicable (non-infectious) diseases (NCDs).

- *Communicable (infectious) diseases:* 'Communicable (infectious) diseases are those diseases for which biological agents or their products are the cause and that are transmissible from one individual to another. The disease process begins when the agent is able to lodge and grow within the body of the host. The process of lodgement and growth of a microorganism or viruses in the host is called infection. Communicable diseases remain an important concern for communities' (Coe, 1970). 'Of the 9.2 million cases of TB that occur in the world every year, nearly 1.9 million are in India accounting for one-fifth of the global TB cases. Experts estimate that about 2.5 million persons have HIV infection in India, world's third highest. More than 1.5 million persons are infected with Malaria every year. Diseases such as dengue and chikungunya have emerged in different parts of India, and a population of over 300 million is at risk of getting acute encephalitis syndrome/Japanese encephalitis. One-third of global cases infected with filaria live in India. Nearly half of leprosy cases detected in the world in 2008 were contributed by India. More than 300 million episodes of acute diarrhoea occur every year in India in children younger than 5 years of age' (MoHFW, 2010: 14).

- *Non-communicable (non-infectious) diseases:* Non-communicable (non-infectious) conditions and diseases are second only to communicable diseases in terms of their contribution to the disease burden in India. These conditions include cardiovascular diseases, cancers, diabetes, respiratory diseases, and mental health diseases. In fact non-communicable (non-infectious) diseases are those that cannot be transmitted from an infected person to another, healthy one.

Report of the National Commission on Macroeconomics and Health (NCMH, 2005) mentions that certain non-cardiovascular diseases will grow from 380 lakh in the year 2005 to 641 lakh in 2015. Diabetes is also emerging as an important health condition in India, with an estimation 310 lakh cases in 2005. The diabetes load is expected to go up to approximately 460 lakh by 2015. Cancers have been attributed to 3.3 per cent of the disease burden in India and approximately 9 per cent of all mortalities. Cancers of the cervix and the breast will continue to have the highest prevalence among cancers of females in India. Tobacco use which is associated with a number of major diseases, including cancers and heart and lung diseases, is prevalent among more than 50 per cent men in India (NFHS–3, 2006), with the highest proportion belonging to the lowest wealth quintile (22%). Mental health disorders are also on the rise, with approximately 650 lakh people in India requiring interventions of mental health. Respiratory diseases such as chronic pulmonary disease (COPD) and asthma are also of significance, with an estimated 1.5 crore chronic cases of asthma in 2001 in India. The increase is as per estimated projections. Analyses by the NCMH indicates that while there is limited evidence on the risk of NCD by economic status, the rural poor will face the threats of these conditions over time, particularly in the absence of any risk protection mechanisms. The current and projected estimates of NCDs by NCMH are presented in Table 1.

Table 1 Diseases burden estimation, 2005

Non-communicable conditions	*Estimate of cases/lakh*	*Projected number (2015) of cases/lakh*
Cancers	8.07 (2004)	9.99
Diabetes	310	460
Mental Health	650	800
Blindness	141.07	129.96
CVDs	290 (2001)	640
COPD and Asthma	405.20 (2001)	596.36

Source: NCMHR (2005) by the Ministry of Health and Family Welfare, Government of India, p. 28, and WHO (Health Systems Development Primary Health Care Current Health Challenges).

Among the other non-communicable diseases, blindness and deafness are major problems. As per survey conducted in 2006–07, the estimated prevalence of blindness has come down to 1 per cent as compared to prevalence of 1.48 per cent found in 1986–89. As per WHO estimates in India, there are approximately 63 million people who are suffering from significant auditory impairment; this places the estimated prevalence of significant hearing loss in India at 6.3 per cent. An even larger percentage of Indian population suffers from milder degrees of hearing loss and unilateral (one sided) hearing loss. These non-communicable diseases are caused by various factors such as genetic, biological, chemical, and social factors such as one's choice of occupation, recreational activities, and living arrangements; poor choice in life can increase one's risk factors which is detrimental to one's health.

Agents of Disease

According to Park (2009), disease 'agent' is defined as a substance, living or non-living, or a force, tangible or intangible, the excessive presence or relative lack of which may initiate or perpetuate a disease process. A disease may have a single agent, a number of independent alternative agents, or a complex of two or more factors whose combined presence is essential for the development of disease. Disease agents may be classified broadly into following groups:

1. *Biological agents:* These are living agents of disease, namely, viruses, fungi, bacteria, protozoa, and metazoa. These agents exhibit certain 'host-related' biological properties such as (i) infective: this is the ability of an infectious agent to invade and multiply in a host, (ii) pathogenicity: this is the ability to induce clinically apparent illness, and (iii) virulence: this is defined as the proportion of clinical cases resulting in severe clinical manifestations. The case fatality rate is one way of measuring virulence.
2. *Nutrient agents:* These can be fats, proteins, carbohydrates, vitamins, minerals, and water. Any excess of deficiency of the intake of nutrient elements may result in nutritional disorders. Protein energy malnutrition (PEM), anaemia, goitre, obesity, and vitamin deficiencies are some of the current nutritional problems in many countries.
3. *Physical agents:* Exposure to excessive heat, cold, humidity, pressure, radiation, electricity, sound, etc., may result in illness.
4. *Chemical agents:* (i) Endogenous: some of the chemicals may be produced in the body as a result of derangement of function, e.g., urea (uraemia), serum bilirubin (jaundice), ketones (ketosis), uric acid (gout), calcium carbonate (kidney stones), etc.: (ii) Exogenous: Agents arising outside human host, for example, allergens, metals, fumes, dust, gases, insecticides, etc. These may be acquired by inhalation, ingestion, or inoculation.
5. *Mechanical agents:* Exposure to chronic friction and other mechanical forces may result in crushing, tearing, sprains, dislocations, and even death.
6. *Social agents:* It is also necessary to consider the social agents of disease. These are poverty, smoking, abuse of drugs and alcohol, unhealthy lifestyles, social isolation, and maternal deprivation.

Cost of Illness and Disease

Segel (2006), quoting from different sources, state: 'A comprehensive cost-of-illness study includes both direct and indirect costs, although the specific focus of a study may make one or the other unnecessary. Direct costs measure the opportunity cost of resources used for treating a particular illness, whereas indirect costs measure the value of resources lost due to a particular illness. Opportunity cost, in this case, is defined by Hodgson and Meiners (1982) as 'the value of the forgone opportunity to use in a different way those resources that are used or lost due to illness'. Although some studies also include intangible costs of pain and suffering, usually in the form of quality of life measures, this category of costs is often omitted because of the difficulty in accurately quantifying it in monetary terms. In such a case, the study should note that intangible costs have been omitted' (Segel, 2006: 4).

Cost of illness (CoI) studies attempt to measure the economic consequences of poor health. A standardized protocol has evolved for CoI studies and Segel, 2006 talks about three components:

(i) Direct Costs

Direct costs refer to health sector costs for prevention, diagnosis, and treatment of diseases and may include costs for ambulance, inpatient, nursing home, outpatient, rehabilitation, allied health, research, community health and medical services, and consumption of pharmaceuticals. Direct costs relate to the resources for which investments are made, whether they are paid or not. So direct medical costs relate to the value of all resources that are employed in the health care system, including informal care, because these resources are directly involved in the process of caregiving, such as prevention, diagnostics, treatment, rehabilitation, and nursing. Direct costs may also include non-health care costs such as travelling costs paid by patients.

When measuring direct costs, studies often measure total direct costs (i.e., the costs of resources used) rather than net direct costs, which subtracts future medical costs avoided because of the death of a patient from total costs. Direct medical costs include hospital inpatient, physician inpatient, physician outpatient, emergency department outpatient, nursing home care, hospice care, rehabilitation care, specialists' and other health professionals' care, diagnostic tests, prescription drugs and drug sundries, and medical supplies. One challenge with calculating direct medical costs, particularly hospital costs, is that charges are often the only data available. Because of the nature of determining hospital charges, they often do not accurately reflect the underlying costs. Charges are often higher than costs to cover losses from patients who are unable to fully pay their expenses, such as procedures not covered by insurance companies, and to cover the rising costs of replacing and updating medical equipment (Segel, 2006).

Non-medical direct costs include transportation costs to health care providers; relocation expenses; and costs of making changes to one's diet, house, car, or related items. However, some non-medical direct costs are generally not included in cost-of-illness studies, such as research, training, and capital costs (e.g., construction). It can be difficult to attribute these costs to a particular disease. Additionally, training health care providers for a particular illness or capital costs, such as a new wing or equipment to treat an illness, is often reflected in the charges of care. To include them separately would lead to the double counting of costs. The specific purpose of the study or the data available may preclude the calculation of non-medical direct costs. When calculated, the focus is often on direct financial costs because non-monetary costs can be difficult to capture.

(ii) Indirect Costs

Indirect costs represent the other portion of estimated costs. Indirect costs of disease are defined as the value of production lost to society due to absence from work and disability and death. These include mortality costs; morbidity costs due to absenteeism and presenteeism; informal care costs (in terms of the opportunity cost of hiring outside care); and, for the few relevant cases such as substance use or violence, losses due to crime (e.g., incarceration, policing, legal, and costs to victims of crime). Indirect costs measure the value of human life or the lost productivity potential of patients who are too ill to work or die prematurely. Society loses some or all of the productive benefit of an ill person and conversely enjoys that benefit if the illness is prevented or the patient cured.

There are important and debatable issues in the measurement of indirect costs. Examples include the use of 'average weekly earnings' as an appropriate measure of a person's productive value and the use of an imputed value for non-marketed production such as unpaid household services. Indirect costs consist of investments indirectly related to the disease and also to resources that are lost or assumed to be lost due to the disease. These costs refer to, for instance, costs of specialized schools for children with intellectual disabilities and judicial costs of criminals with mental disorders.

Indirect costs represent the value of output lost due to illness or premature death. Indirect costs bear a more implicit relation to illness because they do not directly influence expenditures from treating disease and they are not easily measurable. Nevertheless production losses due to illness and production gains due to health care influence the wealth of society and should therefore be incorporated in economic evaluations of health care programmes. Indirect costs are often substantial compared to direct costs and strongly influence the cost-effectiveness.

There are three primary approaches to estimate indirect costs: the human capital method, the friction cost method, and the willingness to pay method.

(a) Human capital method

The human capital method measures the lost production, in terms of lost earnings, of a patient or a caregiver. For mortality or permanent disability costs, the approach multiplies the earnings lost at each age by the probability of living to that age. The earnings in future years are discounted and often a 1 per cent real annual growth rate in earnings is assumed. The human capital approach often includes the value of household work, usually valued as the opportunity cost of hiring a replacement from the labour market.

(b) Friction cost method

A related method, the friction cost method, measures only the production losses during the time it takes to replace a worker. This approach assumes that short-term work losses can be made up by an employee and the loss of employee only results in costs in the time it takes a new employee to be hired and trained, known as the friction period.

(c) Willingness to pay method

The willingness to pay approach measures the amount an individual would pay to reduce the probability of illness or mortality. There are various methods of determining an individual's willingness to pay, including surveys, examining the additional wages for jobs with high risks, examining the demand for products that lead to greater health or safety (e.g., seatbelts), and other related methods (for details, see, www.rti.org/pubs/COI_Primer.pdf).

(iii) Intangible Costs

Intangible costs are a category of costs that is nowadays seldom used. These costs refer to items difficult to measure and value in cost terms, for example, pain and suffering, disability, bereavement, and anxiety associated with a treatment. However, parts of intangible costs are actually not costs (i.e., no resources are denied an alternative use), and overall they are often not strictly intangible, as they can actually be valued through quality-of-life measures (through generic or disease-specific instruments to measure quality of life), or willingness-to-pay (an approach that will not be pursued in this technical document) (see, Stephenson, Bauman, Armstrong, Bellew et al., 2000).

Prevention of Illness

According to Ann Wall and Barry Owen (2005), there is considerable overlap between health promotion and illness prevention, the latter is more specific and clinicians have a larger and more clearly defined role. It can take place at three levels: primary, secondary, and tertiary.

Primary Prevention

Primary prevention is the eradication of the disease agent, resulting in fewer new cases occurring. As with health promotion, some of these measures may be directed at the population at large and are sometimes a statutory requirement. Measures to prevent accidents such as the obligation to wear seat belts and crash helmets; laws relating to drinking and driving; child-proof caps on medicines; and motorway crash barriers are examples of primary prevention, as are vaccination and immunization programmes.

Secondary Prevention

Secondary prevention involves early, pre-symptomatic diagnosis of a disease, and the subsequent modification of its natural history. It reduces the number of people suffering from it at a specified time. Specific disease screening (e.g., for breast or cervical cancer, tuberculosis, and Down's syndrome) comes into this category, as do routine surveillance procedures such as:

- antenatal care,
- monitoring pre-school and school-age children, and
- medical examinations on entry to employment and for those in selected occupations, for example, pilots, train/crane drivers.

Some of these measures have fallen victim to financial constraints within the NHS (Bennett, 1997), but there appears to be a growing market for personal health checks in the commercial sector.

Tertiary Prevention

The third level of prevention seeks to minimize the effects of an illness or disability. The objective is to return the individual to as full a state of health and fitness as possible. Examples include care for the elderly, the chronically sick, people with disabilities, and those suffering from AIDS. It means allocating resources to unglamorous parts of the health and social care system and for research in areas which traditionally have not commanded a large share of the research budget.

Prevention and Control Efforts for Communicable and Non-communicable Diseases

From the above we realize that communities are confronted with a number of health problems—communicable and non-communicable diseases, unintentional injuries, violence, and substance abuse problems and so on. Therefore, there is the need of preventive and control measures for controlling and removing these diseases.

Prevention of Communicable Diseases

According to McKenzie, Pinger, and Kotecki, (2005), prevention and control efforts for communicable diseases include primary, secondary, and tertiary approaches. Jenkins (2003) also has explained and defined such approaches.

(i) Primary prevention of communicable diseases

The primary prevention aims at keeping a disease away from ever beginning or a trauma from ever occurring. Examples include immunization, reducing household hazards, motivating abstinence from illegal drugs, and reducing risk factors for heart disease. The primary prevention measures for communicable diseases at the community level include chlorination of the water supply, the inspection of restaurants and retail food markets, immunization programmes that reach all citizens, the maintenance of a well-functioning sewer system, the proper disposal of solid waste, and the control of vectors and rodents. Besides, these measures personal efforts at primary prevention, including hand washing, the proper cooking of food, adequate clothing and housing, the use of condoms, and obtaining all the available immunizations against specific diseases.

(ii) Secondary prevention of communicable diseases

The secondary prevention involves the early detection and intervention against disease before it develops fully. Screening programmes are prime examples of secondary prevention efforts, providing that persons who screen positive for a disease or condition receive prompt and effective intervention. Conducting screening without full follow-up wastes money and creates anxiety and frustration in the community. At the individual level, secondary preventive measures against communicable diseases involve either (1) self-diagnosis or self-treatment with non-prescription medications or home remedies, or (2) diagnosis and treatment with an antibiotic prescribed by a physician. Secondary preventive measures undertaken by the community against infectious diseases are usually aimed at controlling or limiting the extent of an epidemic. Examples include carefully maintaining records of cases and complying with the regulations requiring the reporting of notifiable diseases and investigating cases and contacts—those who may have become infected through close contact with known cases.

(iii) Tertiary prevention of communicable diseases

Tertiary prevention takes place after a disease or injury has occurred. It seeks not only to prevent deterioration and complications from a disease or injury but also to rehabilitate and return the patient to as full physical, mental, and social function as possible. At the individual level, tertiary preventive measures for the control of communicable diseases include convalescence from infection, recovery to full health, and return to normal activity. In some cases, such as paralytic poliomyelitis, returning to normal activity may not be possible even after extensive physical therapy. Tertiary preventive measures at the community level aimed at preventing the recurrence of an epidemic. The proper removal, embalming, and burial of the dead is an example. Tertiary prevention may involve the reapplication of primary and secondary measures in such a way as to prevent further cases. For example, in some countries, such as the Republic of Korea, people with colds or flu wear gauze masks in public to reduce the spread of disease.

Prevention of Non-communicable Diseases

As we have mentioned above, both the individual and the community can contribute substantially to the prevention and control of multi-causation diseases. The community can provide a pro-health environment—physical, economic, and social—in which it becomes easier for individuals to achieve a high level of health. McKenzie, Pinger, and Kotecki (2005) mention about prevention of non-communicable diseases.

(i) Primary prevention of non-communicable diseases

'Primary preventive measures for non-communicable diseases include adequate food and energy supplies, good opportunities for education, employment, and housing and efficient community services. Beyond this foundation, a community should provide health promotion and health education programmes, health and medical services, and protection from environmental and occupational hazards. The individual should take responsibility for eating properly, exercising adequately, maintaining appropriate weight, and avoiding the overuse of alcohol and other drugs. Individuals can also protect themselves from injury by wearing safety belts, safety goggles, and sunscreen lotions' (ibid.: 108).

(ii) Secondary prevention of non-communicable diseases

'At the individual level, secondary prevention responsibilities include personal screenings such as self-examination of breasts or testes (for cancer of these organs), the hemoccult test (for colorectal cancer), and medical screenings, etc. Secondary preventive measures at the community include the provision of mass screenings for chronic diseases, case-finding measures, and the provision of adequate health personnel, equipment, and facilities for the community' (ibid.: 110).

(iii) Tertiary prevention of non-communicable diseases

'Tertiary prevention for the individual often requires significant behavioural or lifestyle changes. Examples include strict adherence to prescribed medications, exercise programmes, and diet. For example, a heart attack patient could receive nutrition education and counselling and be encouraged to participate in a supervised exercise programme, thus maximizing the use of remaining capabilities. This could lead to a resumption of employment and the prevention of a second heart attack. Tertiary preventive measures for a community include adequate emergency medical personnel, services, and facilities to meet the needs of those citizens for whom primary and secondary preventive measures were unsuccessful. Examples include ambulance services, hospitals, physicians and surgeons, nurses, and other allied health professionals. For certain types of non-communicable health problems, such as those involving substance abuse, regular attendance at support group meetings, or counselling sessions, may constitute an important part of a tertiary prevention program' (ibid.: 111–12).

References

Bennett, F. (1997). 'Social Policy Digest', *Journal of Social Policy*, vol. 6, part II, 248

Brym, R.J. and Lie, J. (2007). *Sociology: Your Compass for a New World*, third edition, UK: Thomson Wadsworth.

Cockerham, W.C. and Ritchey, F.J. (1997). *Dictionary of Medical Sociology*, London: Greenwood Press.

Coe, R.M. (1970). *Sociology of Medicine*, New York/London: McGraw-Hill Book Company.

Giddens, A. (2006). *Sociology*, fifth edition, Cambridge: Polity Press.

Health Systems Development Primary Health Care Current Health Challenges. Available online at: http://www.whoindia.org/LinkFiles/Health_Systems_Development_Primary_Health_Care_Current_health_challenges_.pdf.

Hodgson, T.A. and Meiners, M.R. (1982). 'Cost of Illness Methodology: A Guide to Current Practices and Procedures'. Milbank Memorial Fund Quarterly, 60 (3): 429–462.

Jenkins, C.D. (2003). *Building Better Health: A Handbook of Behavioural Change*, Scientific and Technical Publication No. 590, Pan American Sanitary Bureau, Washington, DC.

Kendall, D. (2011). *Sociology in Our Times*, eighth edition, CA,USA: Wadsworth, Cengage Learning.

McKenzie, J.F., Pinger, R.R. and Kotecki, J.E. (2005). *An Introduction to Community Health*, Fifth Edition, London: Jones and Bartlett Publishers.

MoHFW. (2010). *Annual Report to the People on Health*, Government of India, Ministry of Health and Family welfare, September 2010, p. 14.

NCMHR. (2005). *Report of the National Commission on Macroeconomics and Health*, Ministry of Health and Family Welfare, Government of India, p. 28.

Park, K. (2009). *Preventive and Social Medicine* 20th edition, Jabalpur: Banarsidas Bhanot.

Porta, M. (2008). *A Dictionary of Epidemiology*, fifth edition, New York: Oxford, p. 68.

Segel, J.E. (2006). *Cost-of-Illness Studies: A Primer*, RTI International, RTI-UNC Center of Excellence in Health Promotion Economics.

Stephenson, J., Bauman, A., Armstrong, T., Bellew, B., et al. (2000). *The Costs of Illness Attributable to Physical Inactivity in Australia: A Preliminary Study*, Population Health Division Publications, p. 2.

Thomas, R.K. (2002). *Society and Health: Sociology for Health Professionals*, New York: Kluwer Academic Publishers.

Wall, A. and Owen, B. (2005). *Health Policy*, second edition, London/New York: Routledge.

http://davidscottsociology.tripod.com

http://medical-dictionary.thefreedictionary.com/illness+experience

www.palgrave.com/bilton/pdfs/0333_945719_14_cha13.pdf

CHAPTER SEVEN

Medicalization and Demedicalization

As a critique of medicine for being authoritarian and imperialistic, the concept of medicalization emerged from the intellectual and social turmoil of the 1950s and 1960s and the expansion of its conceptual model to the analysis of social ills and attendant policy or a critique of the expanding role of medicine in the social control of deviant behaviour (Cockerham, 2010). According to Peter Conrad (2007), medicalization describes a process by which non-medical problems become defined and treated as medical problems, usually in terms of illness and disorders. According to Bryans Turner (2006), it is defined as the way in which the scientific knowledge of medical science is applied to behaviours or conditions that are not necessarily biological and this concept was developed (originally in the United States) in the early 1970s, associated with the view of medicine as an instrument of social control. 'An illustration of the medicalization as a phenomenon is provided by the condition of alcoholism. Until the middle of the twentieth century, most people viewed alcoholics as morally weak people who are easily tempted by the pleasure of drink. Gradually, however, medical specialists redefined alcoholism so that most people now consider it a disease, rendering individuals 'sick' rather than 'bad'. Similarly, obesity, drug addiction, child abuse, promiscuity, and other behaviours that used to be moral matters are widely defined today as illnesses for which people need help rather than punishment' (Thomas, 2002: 292).

'Medicalization is also seen as the process through which areas of everyday life have come under the purview of medical authority. Medicalization can also be seen as an attempt to provide an alternative interpretation to problems of existence' (Wainwright, 2008: 97). It refers to the increasing influence of medical institutions and the medical profession on aspects of life that previously had not been considered medical issues. For example, disruptive behaviour by children is now more likely to be defined as attention deficit disorder, with drugs being prescribed for its treatment.

Medicalization is now established as a key sociological concept; however, it is difficult to be specific when it entered the social scientific glossary. It seems that the process was first referred to by critics of the growing influence of psychiatry in the 1960s (although these critics did not use the term explicitly), and grew in popularity in the 1970s when linked with the concept of social control. Since then, medicalization has been applied to a whole variety of problems that have come to be defined as medical, ranging from childbirth and the menopause through to alcoholism and homosexuality. Some analysts have suggested that the growth of medical jurisdiction is 'one of the most effective transformations of the last half of the twentieth century in the West'. For nearly four decades, sociologists, anthropologists, historians, bioethicists, physicians, and others have discussed and written about medicalization. These analysts have focused on the specific instances of medicalization, examining the origins, range, and impact of medicalization on society, medicine, patients, and culture. While some have simply examined the development of medicalization, most have taken a somewhat critical or sceptical view of this social transformation (Conrad, 2007).

Medicalization has been a central concept in medical sociology since the early 1970s. Sociologists have studied medicalization since the late 1960s. The first studies focused on the medicalization of deviance, but soon the concept was seen to be applicable to a wide range of human problems that had entered medical. The key to medicalization is definition; that is, a problem is defined in medical terms, described using medical language, understood through the adoption of a medical framework, or 'treated' with a medical intervention.

According to Conrad and Schneider (1980), medicalization can occur on three distinct levels: (1) conceptually when a medical vocabulary is used to define a problem, (2) institutionally when organizations adopt a medical approach to treating a problem in which they specialize, and (3) at the level of doctor-patient interaction when a problem is defined as medical and medical treatment occurs. As these distinctions illustrate, the process often involves physicians and their treatments directly. However, this is not necessarily so, as in the case of alcoholism where the medical profession may be only marginally involved or not involved at all. Peter Conrad and Joseph Schneider in their well-known book *Deviance and Medicalization: From Badness to Sickness* attempted, following Zola, to identify the conditions under which behaviours are medicalized, pointing to a range of social forces, such as the decline of religion, and the entrepreneurial endeavours of pharmaceutical companies. But they also argued that 'medicalisation is not possible without the complicity or willingness of at least some part of the medical profession' adding that 'often there are medical professionals who act as entrepreneurs for medicalisation' (Scott, 2006: 102).

Medicalization is often associated with the control of deviance 'normal life events', and the ways in which deviant behaviours that were once defined as immoral, sinful, or criminal have been given medical meanings. Talcott Parsons, in his extensive writings on medicine in the 1950s and 1960s, had contended that illness constitutes a form of social deviance that needs to be controlled by society and had pointed to medicine's power to determine whether a person, who was behaving as sick, was actually sick or not, and to legitimate their illness. Medicalization of deviance encompasses or includes alcoholism, mental disorders, opiate addictions, eating disorders, sexual and gender difference, sexual dysfunction, learning disabilities, child and sexual abuse, and other areas of human life. Certain common life processes have been medicalized as well, including anxiety and mood, menstruation, birth control, infertility, childbirth, menopause, ageing, and death.

Medicalization is bidirectional (Conrad, 2007) in the sense that there can be both medicalization and demedicalization. Demedicalization is the political and ideological process by which the medical profession loses influence over various aspects of society or, alternatively, the political and ideological process by which the medical profession, as an agent of social control, loses influence over which social problems and behaviours are defined as sickness as opposed to badness (Cockerham and Ritchey, 1997). But the trend in the past century has been towards the expansion of medical jurisdiction. For demedicalization to occur, the problem must no longer be defined in medical terms, and medical treatments can no longer be deemed appropriate interventions. A classic example is masturbation, which in the nineteenth century was considered a disease and worthy of medical intervention but by the mid-twentieth century was no longer seen as requiring medical treatment. Another most frequently mentioned example is 'homosexuality in America which, until 1973, was defined by the American Psychiatric Association (APA) as an illness. After protests and picketing by the gay liberation movement and support from some sympathetic psychiatrists, the APA voted to declassify it as an illness, a decision that was later endorsed in the United Kingdom. As a result, homosexuality became more widely recognized as a lifestyle choice. With the onset of the AIDS epidemic in the 1980s, however, it became partially remedicalized, although in a different form. Overall, the evidence to date is that medicalization is far more common than de-medicalization but it remains important to see it as a two-way process' (Gabe, Bury, and Elson, 2004: 60).

Medicalization is dynamic and frequently can expand in new directions. During the medicalization era, 1940–85, the jurisdiction of medicine expanded dramatically. One visible area of expansion is how ageing men's lives and bodies are increasingly coming under medical jurisdiction. Television programmes about successful ageing, magazine articles about the best therapy for hair loss, and images used to promote the latest erectile dysfunction medication consistently tell men to 'see your doctor'. This movement of ageing from a natural life event to a medical problem in need of treatment is an example of medicalization (Conrad, 2007). Most early sociological studies took a social constructionist tack in investigating the rise of medicalization. The focus was on the creation (or construction) of new medical categories with the subsequent expansion of medical jurisdiction. Studies of the medicalization of hyperactivity, child abuse, menopause, posttraumatic stress disorder, and alcoholism, among others, broadened our understanding of the range of medicalization and its attendant social processes.

Regarding the nature of medicalization, it has been noted earlier that there is no such agreement about its cause. 'Some have argued that the expansion of medical jurisdiction is primarily a consequence of the medical profession exercising its power to define and control what constitutes health and illness in order to extend its professional dominance. Others have considered medicalization to be the result of broader social processes to which doctors are simply responding' (Gabe, Bury, and Elson, 2004: 61). The concept of medicalization came to the attention of a wider audience through the polemical writings of the Austrian refugee and former Catholic priest, Ivan Illich. Illich (1976) offered a forceful critique of modern medicine, claiming that 'the medical establishment has become a major threat to health' and providing a dossier of medicine's adverse effects—the wrongs and harms it has done—through processes of clinical, social, and cultural 'iatrogenesis' or doctor-induced conditions. 'Ivan Illich (1926–2002) in his medical nemesis (1976) promulgated the idea that societies were becoming increasingly medicalized. Doctors were becoming the new priesthood and modern medicine were creating overdependence on technical fixes' (Turner, 2006: 379). Thus, Illich (1976), for example, attributes medicalization to the increasing professionalization and bureaucratization of medical institutions associated with industrialization. For him, the expansion of modern medicine has created a dependence on doctors and taken away people's ability to engage in self-care (Turner, 2006). Illich, who has so far produced the most radical critique of modern or industrialized medicine, argues that death, pain, and sickness are part of being human. All cultures have developed means to help people cope with all three. Indeed health can even be defined as being successful in coping with these realities. Modern medicine has unfortunately destroyed these cultural and individual capacities, launching instead an inhuman attempt to defeat death, pain, and sickness. It has sapped the will of the people to suffer reality. People are conditioned to get things rather than to do them.

Illich used the concept of iatrogenesis, which means 'doctor-caused illness', that is to say 'harm would not have been caused without the medical intervention. Illich argues that the 'damage done by medicine to the health of the individuals and populations is very significant' (Illich, 1993). This aspect of iatrogenesis is referred to as 'clinical' iatrogenesis and Illich cites drug therapies, doctors, or hospitals as the cause of harm (Barry and Yuill, 2002: 29). A second aspect is that of 'social' iatrogenesis, which means the expansion of medicalization into social life means there is a blind belief in medical progress and expertise, and an institutionalisation of medicine as an industry that commodifies and sells health. Those working in the medical establishment and the medical industry promote the consumption of medical products as the only means of realizing people's health expectations. Hence, 'medical practice sponsors sickness ... reinforcing a morbid society that encourages people to become consumers of curative, preventative, industrial and environmental medicine' (Illich, 1976: 42). Consequently, through social iatrogenesis, 'the responsibility for health has been appropriated from individuals by medicine and the medical industry' (Illich, 1976: 49), and people no longer take responsibility for their health problems (Larkin, 2011). The third aspect is that of 'cultural' iatrogenesis, which denotes a dependence on medicine to cure and to care for. Illich argues that cultural iatrogenesis means that people no longer take responsibility for their own health problems and the diagnosis of their symptoms. 'The result of this dependency is a situation of medical nemesis, where the harm caused by medicine is difficult to eliminate except by recourse to further medical intervention, which in itself results in further harm. Illich paints a picture of an inevitable decline into an increasingly unhealthy world, where the provision of health care ultimately has a negative effect on our well-being' (Barry and Yuill, 2002: 29). Furthermore, Illich is of the view that a proportion of new burden of disease is itself the result of medical interventions in favour of people who are or might be sick of this plethora of therapeutic side effects.

Irving Zola (1972) analysed the increasing pervasiveness of medicine in terms of: (1) expansion into more and more areas of life, (2) absolute control over techniques, (3) access to intimate areas of life, and (4) medical involvement in ethical issues. Zola identified four components of the medicalization of society. First, the expansion of what is deemed relevant to the good practice of medicine, arguing that the shift to multicausal models of illness was leading to more and more aspects of a person's life becoming relevant to their illness—with medicine exploring these wider aspects in order to diagnose and treat illness, and also to prevent it. Second, medicine's absolute control over certain procedures, particularly treatments such as surgery and drugs, permitted the extension of medicine well beyond the diagnosis and treatment of organic disease, as with cosmetic surgery or the prescription of many psychotropic medicines. Third, medicine's absolute access to certain 'taboo' areas—the inner workings of our bodies and minds—meant that anything that could be shown to affect either body or mind could be declared an illness: for instance, the increased in number of people who are consulting doctors to deal with personal problems, alcoholism, and drug addiction. Fourth, medicine was increasingly deemed to be relevant to the 'good practice of life' and so had greater authority to tell people how to live their lives (Scott, 2006).

Zola (1972), too, has argued that medicalization is rooted in the development of an increasingly complex technological and bureaucratic system and a reliance on the expert. Therefore, many writers tend to conceive medicalization in a negative way, focusing on how the phenomenon has resulted in a form of medical social control that serves particular interests in society, or in other words we can say that since health has become a 'paramount value' in society, the sphere of medicine inevitably assumes significance as an institution of social control. 'For Marxists, such medicalization is best seen as serving the interests of the ruling capitalist class. From this standpoint, the creation and manipulation of consumer dependence on medicine are merely examples of a more general dependence upon consumer goods propagated by that class. For feminists, the focus has tended to be on how a male-dominated medical profession (as a result of patriarchal system) has increasingly defined women's problems in medical terms and advocated medical interventions'(Gabe, Bury, and Elson, 2004: 61). This is manifested in studies of reproduction and birth control, childbirth, infertility, premenstrual syndrome, foetal alcohol syndrome, eating disorders, sexuality, menopause, cosmetic surgery, anxiety, and depression. Feminist criticisms, such as the British sociologist Ann Oakley in the book *The Captured Womb* (1984), have accused a medicalized system of ignoring women's own preferences and experiences. In other contexts, women are similarly seen as the object of patriarchal medical control, for instance over drugs (especially the prescription of tranquillizers) and surgery, and in general the treatment of women within the medical system is accused of serving to enforce passivity and dependence.

Peter Conrad (2007) incisively examined the particular gendered aspects of medicalization. 'Scholarly examinations of gender and medicalization, which have largely focused on the medicalization of women, have generally ignored the medicalization of men's lives. Some have argued that men are not as vulnerable to medicalization as are women: the substantial literature on the medicalization of childbirth, premenstrual syndrome, menopause, and anorexia in women clearly shows that more of women's life experiences are medicalized than men's. One of several reasons analysts typically give for women's vulnerability to medicalization is the traditional definition of a healthy body. On the one hand, Alan Petersen notes, male bodies have been constructed through scientific and cultural practices as naturally different from female bodies, and the bodies of White, European, middle-class, heterosexual men have been constructed as the standard for measuring and evaluating other bodies. On the other hand, Riessman suggests that women are more vulnerable to medicalization than are men because their physiological processes (menstruation, birth) are visible, their social roles expose them to medical scrutiny, and they are often in a subordinate position to men in the clinical domain' (Conrad, 2007: 24).

Further, 'the major contribution of French social philosopher Foucault to medical sociology is his analysis of the social functions of the medical profession, including the use of medical knowledge as a means of social control and regulation, as he studied madness, clinics, and sexuality. Foucault (1973) found two distinct trends emerging in the history of medical practice: 'medicine of the species' (the classification, diagnosis, and treatment of disease) and 'medicine of social spaces' (the prevention of disease). The former defined the human body as an object of study subject to medical intervention and control, while the latter made the public health subject to medical and civil regulation. The surveillance of human sexuality by the state, church, and medicine subjected the most intimate bodily activities to institutional discourse and monitoring. Thus, bodies themselves came under the jurisdiction of experts on behalf of society' (Cockerham, 2010: 16). Michel Foucault wrote about medicalization in one of his earlier works, *Birth of the Clinic*.

The two dreams (i.e., nationalised medical profession and disappearance of disease) are isomorphic; the first expressing in a very positive way the strict, militant, dogmatic medicalisation of society, by way of a quasi-religious conversion and the establishment of a therapeutic clergy; the second expressing the same medicalisation, but in a triumphant, negative way, that is to say, the volitization of disease in a corrected, organized, and ceaselessly supervised environment, in which medicine itself would finally disappear, together with its object and *raison d'être* (Conrad, 2007: 13).

'Michel Foucault saw medicalization not as the simple exercise of personal power by profession intent on extending its boundaries, but as a historical process deriving from the power of clinical knowledge and the redefinition of medicine to include psychological, economic, and social 'health'' (Turner, 2006: 379). Michel Foucault argued that the dominance of professional power of doctors led to their convergence around the medical gaze, through which the sick are represented as objects for surveillance and technical intervention. 'In a series of books such as *Madness and Civilisation, The Birth of the Clinic*, and *The History of Sexuality*, Foucault emphasized the increasing penetration of medical ideas and practices in Western ways of thinking, particularly from the period of the Enlightenment onwards. However, his conception of power differed from that of writers such as Zola or Illich. In

Foucault's view, power and knowledge are inextricably linked and power operates through the development and construction of discourses. These constitute ways of seeing and understanding the world and are not just constraining but also productive. Medical discourses are guidelines as to how patients should understand and regulate their bodies, and they create new ways of thinking, new possibilities, and new opportunities. According to Foucault, power does not exist in doctors considered as 'figures of domination'. Instead it exists in relationships between people' (Scott, 2006: 102).

Foucault did not typically use the term 'medicalization' but tended to present a consonant vision that shows the impact of medical discourses on people's lives But most studies of medicalization tend to be social constructionist rather than Foucauldian in orientation' (Conrad, 2007: 8). Nikolas Rose has expanded the Foucauldian perspective on biopolitics and offers three phases of biopolitics to understand new forms of medical culture and social control. 'Risk politics characterizes the first half of the twentieth century, when the focus was on prevention of major public health problems. Molecular politics is a reorganization of the medical gaze at the molecular level. This politics is represented by, for example, biological psychiatry, a discipline that looks at the neurotransmitters of the brain to identify chemical imbalances that are seen as the causes of mental pathologies. Current biopolitics has taken the character of ethopolitics: it demands an optimization of one's corporeality to embrace an enlarged will to health and concerns itself with 'the self-techniques by which human beings should judge themselves and act upon themselves to make themselves better than they are'. It is argued that this new regimen blurs the boundaries between expert knowledge and the individual's will to self-regulation. In this kind of society, individuals are still dependent on experts who provide the technologies for rational management of the self' (Cockerham, 2010: 345).

Sociologists have rarely looked at the growth of health care in terms of markets. 'But when medical products, services, or treatments are promoted to consumers to improve their health, appearance, or well-being, we see the development of medical markets. This should not be surprising, given our increasingly corporatized health system and the growing consumer culture for health-related products and services' (Conrad, 2007: 16). Thus, the concept of medicalization has proved a useful descriptive tool for sociologists and other intellectuals and is still used quite frequently, almost invariably with critical force. Some, following Illich, have also been critical of the power medicalization gives the profession and of the ideas and practices of medicine, and some have suggested it is to blame for the power it exercises. These negative views of medicine and of its possible role in medicalization are regarded by others as misplaced or simplistic and this, along with the spread of theoretical ideas such as those of Foucault, may help to account for the fact that the term is now less widely used than formerly. Yet it continues to have value as a descriptive term to highlight an important set of social changes.

Criticisms

Studies of medicalization have not been without controversy. Conrad (2007) has summarized some of these critiques. According to Conrad, these controversies are important to moving the study of medicalization forward. 'The earliest critiques argued that the medicalization case has been overstated and that significant constraints limit rampant medicalization (Fox, 1977; Strong, 1979). Some of these critiques conflated deprofessionalization with demedicalization (Fox, 1977). Others failed to recognize that most studies of medicalization adopt a historical, social-constructionist perspective. From a sociological perspective, case studies of medicalization have created a new understanding of the social process involved in the cultural production of medical categories or knowledge; however, these investigations do not necessarily contain a mandate as to how the categories and knowledge are to be evaluated.

Despite all these criticisms, medicalization remains a useful concept for sociologists of health and illness and there is a need to go beyond the accumulation of different cases of medicalization to try and develop a more integrated theory of the process of medicalization, its causes, and consequences and to relate these to recent changes in medical organization and knowledge and the growing challenge to medical authority.

References

Barry, A.M. and Yuill, C. (2002). *Understanding Health: A Sociological Introduction*, London/Thousand Oaks/New Delhi: Sage Publications.

Cockerham, W.C. (2010). *The New Blackwell Companion to Medical Sociology*, UK: Wiley Blackwell Publication.

Conrad, P. (2007). *The Medicalization of Society: On the Transformation of Human Conditions into Treatable Disorders*, Baltimore, Maryland: Johns Hopkins University Press.

Conrad, P., and Schneider, J.W. (1980). *Deviance and Medicalization: From Badness to Sickness,* Michigan: Mosby.

Foucault, M. (1973). *The Birth of the Clinic: An Archaeology of Medical Perception,* Tavistock Publications. First published by Tavistock Publications Limited in 1973, First published in Routledge Classics in 2003, Oxon

Fox, R.C. (1977). 'The Medicalization and Demedicalization of American Society', *Daedalus,* 106: 9–22

Gabe, J., Bury, M. and Elson, M. (2004). *Key Concepts in Medical Sociology*, London: Sage Publications.

Illich, I. (1976). *Limits to Medicine; Medical Nemesis: The Expropriation of Health*, London: Marion Boyars Publishers.

——. (1993). 'The Epidemics of Modern Medicine', in N. Black, D. Boswell, A. Gray, S. Murphy, and J. Popay, *Health and Disease: A Reader*. Milton Keynes: Open University Press

Larkin, M. (2011). *Social Aspects of Health, Illness and Healthcare*, New York: Open University Press.

Scott, J. (2006). *Sociology: The Key Concepts*, London/New York: Routledge, Taylor and Francis Group.

Strong, P. (1979). 'Sociological Imperialism and the Profession of Medicine: A Critical Examination of the Thesis of Medical Imperialism', *Social Science and Medicine*, 13A: 199–215

Thomas, R.K. (2002). *Society and Health: Sociology for Health Professionals*, New York: Kluwer Academic Publishers.

Turner, B. (2006). *The Cambridge Dictionary of Sociology*, Cambridge: Cambridge University Press.

Zola, I.K. (1972). 'Medicine as an Institution of Social Control'. *The Sociological Review*, 20: 487–504. www.bmj.com/content/324/7342/859.full

Chapter Eight

Systems of Medicine and Medical Pluralism in India

Pluralism is a concept that has been used in many different ways, most notably in relation to social and cultural phenomena. In contrast to monism or unity, the term acknowledges multiplicity and difference and that there are different ways of knowing and being. According to Jonathan Gabe, Mike Bury, and Maryann Elson (2004), medical anthropologists were the first to use the concept of 'medical pluralism'. Having always described different healing practices as part of their study of culture, it is seen during 1980s that medical anthropologists give more specific attention to the collaboration between indigenous/traditional medicine and biomedicine in Latin America, Asia, and Africa. Sarah Cant and Ursula Sharma (1999) say that pluralism in health care is nothing new. There has always been the possibility of choice between different kinds of practitioner, and between consulting and self-prescribing, and there have always been multiple ways of understanding health and sickness. According to Gabe, Bury, and Elson, 'medical pluralism refers to the co-existence in a society of differing medical traditions, grounded in different principles or based on different world-views' (2004: 183).

Veena Bhasin (2007: 9–10) says that 'medical pluralism may be defined as the synchronic existence in a society of more than one medicine systems grounded in different principles or based on different worldviews. Medical pluralism offers a variety of treatment options that health seekers may choose to utilize exclusively, successively, or simultaneously. In most parts of India, multiple therapy systems and a diversity of health behaviour patterns coexist. Health care in India is characterized by medical pluralism, including self-care, consultations with traditional healers and/or primary health care services (PHCs), etc. India, like other traditional societies, has a wealth of medical knowledge. In addition to codified traditional systems—Ayurvedic, Unani, and Siddha, there is ethno-medicine, religious healing, and folk medicine.'

Basically, there are two systems of health care in the developing world: one is traditional and the other is western in derivation. 'Traditional medicine includes all kinds of folk medicine, unconventional medicine, herbal medicine, massage, homeopathy, mud bath, music therapy, wax bath, reflexology, dance therapy, hydrotherapy, mind and spirit therapies, self-exercise therapies radiation and vibration, osteopathy, chiropractics (a system of complementary medicine based on the diagnosis and manipulative treatment of misalignments of the joint, especially those of the spinal column), aromatherapy, preventive medicine, radiant heat therapy, therapeutic fasting and dieting spinal manipulation, psychotherapy, etc., and indeed any kind of therapeutic method that had been handed down by the tradition of a community or ethnic group. In contrast to traditional health care system, the official health care system is based on western science and technology. In keeping with the scientific tradition, its practitioners make every effort to separate themselves from broader social and cultural concerns and influences' (Bhasin, 2007: 10). Indian Medical Council Act formally established the traditional systems—Ayurvedic, Unani, and Siddha—as official components of national health care in India.

Diana Kendall (2011) explains the functional approach on medical pluralism. According to the functionalist approach, if society is to function as a stable system, it is important for people to be healthy so that they can contribute to the proper functioning of their society. In order to maintain themselves in a normal state of health, they use various types of medicines and medical practices. On the other hand, it can be said that during illness the physicians prescribe various medical treatments in order to bring the patients in a normal state of health, so that he can perform his assigned roles in a society.

Indian medical pluralism is characterized by plurality in terms of system of medicine and the forms of practice: Ayurvedic, Unani, Siddha, Allopathic, and Homeopathy (AYUSH) reflect plurality of the system and private as well as government practitioners reflect plurality of the form. The goals of the AYUSH department are the promotion and propagation of the traditional systems of medicine especially in the background of increasing chronic disorders due to modern day lifestyles. In order to meet this commitment, the department of AYUSH has taken steps at all levels in the health care system, improving access to and quality of public health delivery and promoting health and the prevention of diseases (MoHFW, 2010). According to Borins (1987), the majority of Indians—more than 700 million people—still receive medical services from indigenous practitioners who treat their patients according to the principles of three ancient systems of Indian medicine: the Ayurvedic, the Siddha medicine of South India, and the Unani or Graeco-Arabic medicine. Besides these systems of medicine, there are various types of folk and tribal medical beliefs and practices which are often based on magic and sorcery. These practices have existed from times immemorial (Minocha, 1967).

Ayurvedic System of Medicine

India has had a well-developed system of medicine from ancient times known as ayurveda, that is, a science of life or longevity. Ayurveda is an integral part of the Vedas, which makes it at least 5,000 years old. According to Filliozat (1964: 1), Ayurveda is '... sometimes considered as a secondary part (*upanga*) of the Atharvaveda and sometimes as a secondary Veda (*upaveda*) of the Rig-Veda' (Minocha, 1967). Ayurvedic practitioners are similar to practitioners of the Unani and Siddha systems, since they use diet, herbs, minerals, colour, germs, yoga, and pranayama (scientific breathing techniques used in treating patients); they also consider exercise, life habits, seasons of the year, and individual temperament into consideration. They also classify foods according to temperature and give hot foods for certain problems and cold foods for others. They gather these foods from neighbouring gardens and forests and prepare the medicines for their patients themselves or under their own supervision. In this way, they ensure the purity of drugs and preparation they used.

Ayurveda philosophy believes that each human being is a sum total of five basic gross elements (*pancha mahabhutas*), seven body tissues (*sapta dhatus*), and five senses (*panchedriyas*) along with mind (*manas*), which performs the sensory and motor functions, intellect (*buddhi*), and soul (*atma*). The pancha mahabhutas are lithosphere (solid earth), hydrosphere (water in various forms), atmosphere (air), sunlight (fire or energy), and ether (space). Together these create three humours in human body called *tridoshas.* So as long as three *doshas* are in balance, body will be healthy. Imbalance among *doshas* appears in the form of various kinds of diseases.

Unani Medicine

More than anyone else it was Hippocrates (460 BC) who laid the foundations of the Unani medicine. The Unani medicine owes its origin, as its name suggests to Greece (Yunnan). From Greece it travelled to Arabia and then to Persia and Indian systems of medicine. The Unani system of medicine is very close to India's Ayurvedic system. India recognizes it as one of the indigenous system of medicine. The Unani system is based on the humoral theory. Humoral theory believes that there are four types of body fluids: the dam (blood—is hot and moist), balgam (phlegm—is cold and moist), safra (yellow bile—is hot and dry), and saoda (black bile—is cold and dry). Each of these is linked to its own temperament (Mishra, 2007).

Borins (1987) says that the Unani system places great reliance on the pulse for diagnosis. Unani practitioners in India have started to use modern techniques such as microscopic examination, chemical analysis, radiography, and electrocardiography for treating patients. In the Unani system, the treatment may involves: (a) regional therapy, which includes massage therapy, physical exercise, and cupping, (b) dietotherapy, which includes treating certain elements by administration of specific diets or by regulating the quality or quantity of food, and (c) pharmacotherapy, which includes the use of natural drugs obtained from plants, herbs, minerals, and animal parts. Thus, the Unani practitioners in India treat their patients by using regional therapy, dietotherapy, and pharmacotherapy.

Siddha System of Medicine

Siddha system of medicine is another type of medicine used by the Indians during their illness or disease. The Siddha system is based on the principle of free flow of pranic energy (life) all through the body all the time. When this flow stopped, diseases take their roots. Restoring the free flow of energy is restoration of the health of the patient. No medicines are needed for this. It can be done by meditation and yoga is used for treatment. The Siddha practitioners mostly examine the patients tongue, nails, eyes, and lips.

Folk Medicine

A relatively modern term, folk medicine means the care of the sick by unlicensed healers mostly including those who practice herbal and magical medicine. It is a body of knowledge distinct from modern and scientific medicine but may coexist in the same Indian culture (Bhasin, 2007). Folk medicine is diverse, ecosystem and ethnic community specific (Gangadharan and Shankar, 2009: 181). It is an oral tradition purely empirical in nature that exists in all rural communities throughout India. Herbal medicine is one aspect of folk medicine which is also used by the people of India, which involves the use of parts of the gathered plant to make teas, poultices, or powders that purportedly effect cures. *Vaata*, *pittaa*, *vaayu*, *kapha*, *ushna*, and *sheetala* are the technical terms that are used by folk healers and traditional practitioners. All these terms form part of the knowledge of folk practitioners and the households. The classical text of Ayurveda also mentions about the folk traditions and healers.

Yoga Therapy

H.K. Bakhru (2010) says that the term 'yoga' is derived from the Sanskrit root '*yug*' which means 'to join'. It signifies the union between individual soul (*jivatma*) and the universal soul (*parmatma*). The yoga aims at obtaining relief from pain and suffering. Yoga therapy is a specialized form of yogic culture. Yoga therapy refers to the treatment of diseases by means of exercises, which may be physical and mental or both. This mode of treatment has been practiced in India from very ancient times. In India, the yogic *kriyas*, *asanas*, and *pranayma* constitute the physical basis of yoga. The practice of *kriyas* and *asanas* helps people in excellent circulation and also energizes and stimulates their major endocrine glands of the body. Yogic exercises promote inner health and harmony and its regular practice helps to prevent and cure many common ailments. Tensions, that is, physical, mental, or emotional, can be eliminated by doing yogic exercises. Similarly, *pranayma* slows down the ageing process. In *pranayma*, the breathing rate is slowed down to ones or twice a minute and the breath inhaled is deep and full, taking nearly 100 cubic inches of air.

Faith Healing

For centuries people claiming powers to relieve pain and sufferings had an important place in society. Not only illiterate people but also educated people with scientific backgrounds have some faith in the powers of these healers. Healers may chant some *mantras* given to them by some saint or *fakir* to ward off the evil, and some healers cure people by touching the affected parts of the body. In order to get recovery from the ailments, a number of people in India visit temples, *durgahs,* churches, and other religious places. These people usually develop a strong faith in the power of the deity. In the recent past, faith healing has emerged in a different and very sophisticated form which attracted educated people, and people suffering from systematic disorders and incurable diseases are attracted most. However, the fact does remain that as the faith of the people in modern allopathic medicines declines, the popularity of the faith healing increases (Mishra, 2007).

Modern (Allopathic) Medicine

The allopathic or 'modern' or 'western' system of medicine entered India with the British. Allopathic medicine refers to the practice of conventional medicine that uses pharmacologically active agents or physical interventions to treat or suppress symptoms of diseases or conditions. Modern medicine approaches health care from two angles. The first, the medical model, focuses on the eradication of illness through diagnosis and effective treatment. The second, the social model, focuses on changes in society and in people's own lifestyles to make the population healthier. It is increasingly widespread and more widely accepted than other forms of medicine. Modern medicine is notably secular, indifferent to ideas of the supernatural or the spirit, and concentrates on the body and society to determine causes and cures. Modern (allopathic) medicine consists of two new branches of medicines:

(a) *Curative medicine:* Curative medicine aims at removing diseases from patients. Curative medicine involves treatment by administering antibacterial and antibiotic drugs, which produce a reaction that neutralizes the disease. It is as old as medicine itself but in the twentieth century it acquired unprecedented scientific knowledge about diseases, medicines, and ways of administering the medicines. As a result of this specialization, surgery, radiology, and anaesthesia are developed, which are based on skills. No doubt, specialization has raised the standards of medical care but the cost of the medical services has increased manyfold. Today it is difficult for a poor person to secure medical services at a price he can afford.

(b) *Preventive medicine:* Preventive medicine developed as a branch of medicine distinct from public health. By definition, preventive medicine is applied to health of persons in groups, that is, it focuses on population rather than individuals. Primary objective of preventive medicines is the prevention of diseases and promotion of health. Preventive medicines have helped us in decreasing the rate of morbidity and mortality caused from diphtheria, tetanus, typhoid, fever, and other diseases. In the field of nutrition, preventive medicine has played a very important role. Nutritional blindness and iodine deficiency disorders have been reduced substantially. Discovery of vitamins, minerals, proteins, and other nutritional requirements of a healthy body has prevented the attack of many diseases. Population control through fertility control and contraceptives is the latest addition to the responsibilities of preventive medicine. Modern preventive medicine has been defined as the art and science of health promotion, disease prevention, disability limitation, and rehabilitation. It operates at three levels. At the primary level, it aims at keeping people healthy and immune from disease; at the secondary level, it treats those who are suffering from disease; and at the tertiary level, it tries to lower the impact of the disease on those who have it (see, Mishra, 2007; Park, 2009).

Social Medicine

Social medicine emerged in the nineteenth century as a movement to investigate medical problems in the light of social science. Social medicine is the epidemiological study of people and community, rather than individuals. According to Park (2009), social medicine is the study of a man as a social being in his total environment. It is concerned with all the factors affecting the distribution of health and ill health in populations, including the use of health services. In India, it is still an academic discipline something like medical geography.

Thus, the concept of medical pluralism has, through use, come to be associated with the coexistence of biomedicine and alternative medicine. However, its descriptive potential is much wider than this, encompassing the idea of differences within and across healing systems. The conceptual and applied development of this concept will mean that it continues to have strong and adaptive relevance for medical sociology or sociology of health.

References

Bakhru, H.K. (2010). *A Complete Handbook of Nature Cure*, Mumbai: Jaico Publishing.

Bhasin, V. (2007). *Medical Anthropology: A Review*, Delhi: Department of Anthropology, University of Delhi.

Borins, M. (1987). 'Traditional Medicine in India'. Can. Fam. Physician, April. vol. 33, Available online at http://www.ncbi.nlm.nih.gov/pmc/articles/PMC2218447/

Cant, S. and Sharma, U. (1999). *A New Medical Pluralism*, London/New York: Routledge Publications.

Filliozat, J. (1964). *The Classical Doctrine of Indian Medicine*, New Delhi: Munshiram Manoharlal.

Gabe, J., Bury, M. and Elson, M. (2004). *Key Concepts in Medical Sociology*, London: Sage Publications.

Gangadharan, G.G. and Shankar, D. (2009). 'Medical Pluralism: The Challenges Ahead', *Indian Journal of Traditional Knowledge*, 8(2): 181.

Kendall, D. (2011). *Sociology in Our Times*, eighth edition, CA, USA: Wadsworth, Cengage Learning.

Minocha (Ahluwalia), A. (1967). 'Sociology of Medicine in India: An Approach', *Economic and Political Weekly*, 2(22): 1007–1012.

Mishra, R.P. (2007). *Geography of Health*, Delhi: Concept Publications.

MoHFW. (2010). *Annual Report to the People on Health*, GoI, Ministry of Health and Family Welfare (MoHFW), New Delhi.

Park, K. (2009) *Preventive and Social Medicine* 20th edition, Jabalpur: Banarsidas Bhanot.

Chapter Nine

Widening Dimensions of Health and Determinants of Health

Health finds different interpretations from different perspectives. The biomedical approach, which dominated the medical thought till the end of nineteenth century and based on the 'germ theory of disease', views health as an 'absence of diseases'. This approach almost ignores the role of environmental, psychological, and other socio-cultural factors in defining health. The ecological approach views health as a dynamic equilibrium between man and his environment. For them, disease is maladjustment of the human organism to environment. The psychological approach states that health is not only related to body but also to mind and especially to the attitude of the individual. The socio-cultural approach considers health as a product of the social and community structure (see Advani and Akram, 2007).

Health

Health is man's natural condition; health is his birth right. It is the result of living in accordance with natural laws pertaining to the body, mind, and environment. These laws relate to fresh air, sunlight, diet, exercise, rest and relaxation, sleep, cleanliness, right attitude of mind, good habits, and above all lifestyle. The WHO definition of health states that health is a state of complete physical, mental, and social well-being, and not merely an absence of disease or infirmity. Health is multidimensional; three important dimensions of health are reflected in the WHO definition which are physical, mental, and social (Park, 2005).

- *Physical dimension:* The state of physical health implies the notion of 'perfect functioning' of the body. It conceptualizes a state in which every organ is in perfect harmony with the rest of body. The signs of physical health in an individual are as follows: a good complexion, a clean skin, bright eyes, lustrous hair with a body well clothed with firm flesh, not too fat, a sweet breath, a good appetite, sound sleep, and easy and coordinated movements.
- *Mental dimension:* Good mental health is the ability to respond to the many varied experiences of life with flexibility and a sense of purpose. The signs of a mentally healthy person are as follows: he is free from internal conflicts, he is well-adjusted, and he has a good self-control. Further, he is not overcome by emotions; he is not dominated by fear, anger, jealousy, guilt, or worries; he faces problems and solves them intelligently.
- *Social dimension:* The social dimension of health includes the levels of social skills one possesses, social functioning, and the ability to see oneself as a member of a large society. In general, social health takes into account that every individual is a part of a family and of wider community and focuses on social and economic conditions and well-being of the 'whole person' in the context of his social network

Holistic Approach to Health

The basic concept of holistic health is that a human being should be an integrated whole. Health professionals keep refining their definition of health to describe a state of total well-being. The constant interaction between all elements of the body makes it impossible to separate mental health from physical health, social well-being from spiritual well-being, or any one of these elements from the others. Each contributes to the status of the others.

According to this total concept, better known as holistic concept, a healthy person is one who successfully experiences growth and development in all of these elements more or less at the same time.

Frazer Brockington identifies five stages in the preservation of health. The most important idea is the promotion of health by positive vital forces that is by teaching physiological principles of healthy living or by providing good diet. The second stage seeks to prevent illness, chiefly by the application of medical knowledge in relation to a specific disease by inoculation, etc. The third seeks to detect early departure from normal health with the object of bringing about a remedy, in advance for the established diseases. The fourth stage constitutes after care of sickness or injury in which remedies are sought for social factors, and the last stage deals with the management of incurable sickness and it seeks for a worthwhile amelioration of it (Hobson, 1965).

Responsibility for Health

The health status of an individual, a community, or a nation is determined by the interplay and integration of two ecological universes, the internal environment of the man himself, and the external environment which surrounds him. 'Health is on one hand a highly personal responsibility and on the other hand a major public concern. It involves the joint efforts of the whole social fabric, namely, the individual, the community, and the state to protect and promote health' (Park, 2005: 20). The individual responsibility for health largely depends upon self-care, which refers to those health-generating activities that are undertaken by the persons themselves. It comprises observance of simple rules of behaviour relating to diet, sleep, exercise, weight, hygiene, and the overall lifestyle. It also includes undertaking measures for preventing disease, treatment during illness, and remaining aware about the biomedical and mental-psychological conditions of the individual concerned.

The responsibility for health does not end with the individual and community effort. In all modern societies, the state assumes responsibility for health and welfare of its people. The Constitution of India, in the Directive Principles of State Policy, asserts that health is a state responsibility. The fundamental right of 'right to life', as ensured by Article 21 of the Constitution, also makes it binding for the government to ensure proper living condition for its citizen. The Government of India has a health policy of its own and consistently designs it to meet the health requirements of its people. Responsibility for health of the individuals is also shared by international agencies. The health of mankind requires the cooperation of governments, the people, and national and international organizations both within and outside the United Nations system in achieving universal health goals.

Widening Dimensions of Health

It is customary to distinguish between both negative and positive definitions of health and functional and experiential definitions (Calnan, 1987). The biomedical view of health—the absence of disease—is clearly negative. By contrast, the comprehensive definition given by World Health Organization (WHO)—health is a state of complete physical, mental, and social well-being—is positive. A functional definition implies the ability to participate in normal social roles, and this may be contrasted with an experiential definition that takes sense of self into account (Kelman, 1975). Further, McKenzie, Pinger, and Kotecki (2002) have defined health as a dynamic state or condition that is multidimensional in nature and results from person's adaptations to his/her environment. It is a resource for living and exists in varying degrees.

We also need to understand the meaning of illness because in contemporary paradigms, we talk about health and illness together. Kleinman (1988: 3) suggests that disease is a biophysical event and the prime concern of medical practitioners, whereas illness 'refers to how the sick person and members of the family or wider social network perceive, live with and respond to symptoms and disability'. Dingwall (1976: 26) argues that there is no such thing as 'essential illness', rather, illness is construed through the meanings and interpretations that are accorded to certain categories of experience and 'there is no necessary relationship to any biological happening'. According to Giddens (2006), illness has both personal and public dimensions. When we become ill, not only do we experience pain, discomfort, confusion, and other challenges, but others are affected as well. Hence, Sarah Nettleton (1995: 78) concludes, 'rather than simply observing illness behaviour, sociologists must endeavour to understand illness action. The former refers to the way people behave given the presence of symptoms, whilst the latter focuses on how people make sense of and interpret their illness experience and, crucially, what it means to them' (see, Akram, 2012b).

The Determinants of Health

Many factors combine to affect the health of individuals and communities. Whether people are healthy or not is determined by their circumstances and environment. To a large extent, factors such as where we live, the state of our environment, genetics, our income and education level, and our relationships with friends and family all have considerable impacts on health, whereas the more commonly considered factors such as access and use of health care services often have less of an impact. Health determinants can be categorized as: personal behaviour and lifestyles; influences within communities which can sustain or damage health; living and working conditions and access to health services; and general socio-economic, cultural, and environmental conditions.

The context of people's lives determines their health, and so blaming individuals for having poor health or crediting them for good health is inappropriate. Individuals are unlikely to be able to directly control many of the determinants of health. These determinants—or things that make people healthy or not—include the above factors, and many others, which are as follows:

- *Income and social status*: Higher income and social status are linked to better health. The greater the gap between the richest and poorest people, the greater the differences in health. Poverty creates serious handicaps in the path of good health.
- *Education*: Low education levels are linked with poor health, more stress, and lower self-confidence. In the case of health of infant and children, mother's education is very important. Health education and awareness is also a great facilitator in the prevention of communicable diseases.
- *Physical environment*: Clean air, healthy workplaces, safe houses, communities, and roads all contribute to good health. Employment and working conditions—people in employment,

particularly those who have more control over their working conditions, are healthier. Hazardous work situation creates occupational disease.

- *Social support networks*: Greater support from families, friends, and communities is linked to better health. Culture, customs and traditions, and the beliefs of the family and community all affect health. Social and cultural capitals are important health inputs.
- *Genetics*: Inheritance plays a part in determining lifespan, healthiness, and the likelihood of developing certain illnesses or immunity. Personal behaviour and coping skills—balanced eating, keeping active, smoking, drinking, and how we deal with life's stresses and challenges—all affect health. However, social factors do have a long-term impact on the genetic factors also.
- *Health services*: Availability, accessibility, acceptability, and affordability of health services and other related determinants of health that prevent occurrence of disease and treat disease are also important determinants. In contemporary world, health care services are indispensable for health.
- *Age and gender*: Men and women have different health requirements at different stages. Hence, age and gender are also important health determinants.
- *Lifestyle*: Lifestyle is increasingly being considered as an important determinant of health. Diseases such as obesity or diabetes are also related to food habits and lifestyle. They are also depended on level of physical activity maintained in the changing lifestyles patterns. Smoking or consumption of tobacco is a cause of cancer in various parts of the world.
- *Biological agents*: Biological organisms such as bacteria and virus play the role of carrier of infection. Such factors prevail under specific conditions. Prevalence level of such factors also play important role in ensuring health conditions of population.
- *Basic health goods*: Food, nutrition, potable water, and sanitation are the foundation stone of health and can be categorized as basic health goods (BHGs). Availability, accessibility, and affordability of these BHGs are important for having good health in the society.

Social Determinants of Health

The High Level Expert Group (HLEG, 2011), which was constituted by Government of India in 2011 for suggesting the model of Universal Health Coverage (UHC) for its citizen, has made several recommendations for universal health coverage for its people. Besides, it has made observations on the prevailing health conditions in India. It has noted specific findings related to social determinants of health in India. The vision of the HLEG is based on the World Health Organization's Commission on Social Determinants of Health (CSDH) (WHO, 2005, 2010). The CSDH embedded the goal of universal health care in strategies that include improving daily living conditions, tackling the inequitable distribution of money, power, and resources, as well as measuring and understanding health inequities. The CSDH defines the Social Determinants of Health (SDH) as 'the conditions in which people are born, grow, live, work and age, including the health system'. It encourages countries to provide Universal Health Coverage to address health inequity directly. The report acknowledges, moreover, that health inequities arise not only from within but also from beyond the domain of health, through other social determinants, including the 'unequal distribution of power, income, goods, and services, globally and nationally, the consequent unfairness in the immediate, visible circumstances of people's lives—their access to health care, schools, and education, their conditions of work and leisure, their homes, communities, towns, or cities—and their chances of leading a flourishing life'. It is already well established that among the most critical social determinants of health is the health system itself.

In India, the movement towards Universal Health Coverage (UHC) will necessitate reform of the health system. In addition, Universal Health Coverage will only be possible if there is accompanying action on social determinants such as food and nutrition security, social security, water and sanitation, work and income security as well as social inclusion and equity across gender, caste, and religious categories. In addition, macroeconomic policies in the country will also have a significant bearing on Universal Health Coverage. The HLEG (2011) report also examines the rationale for a social determinant perspective in Indian context and it is briefly presented here:

The Rationale for a Social Determinants Perspective in the Indian Context

According to the HLEG (2011), the need for action on social determinants emerges from the recognition that there are huge differentials among and between classes and castes, gender gaps and wide regional variations in both disease burden and response by the health system and others concerned with development.

(a) Nutrition and Food Security

More than a fourth of the world's population who are hungry are Indians. As per the WHO's standards, 40 per cent of Indian children under the age of three are underweight, 45 per cent are stunted, and 23 per cent have wasting. Malnutrition itself is the result of several other determinants that have extended and extenuating lifetime impact on the health and well-being of women and their children.

Even economically developed states—Gujarat, Maharashtra, Andhra Pradesh, and Karnataka—have high levels of food insecurity. As per the New Delhi Birth Cohort, the population attributable to risk of being underweight is 28 per cent for six month olds, as compared to 18 per cent among five year olds—clearly the concentration of nutrition-related morbidity follows a reverse age gradient, rendering the youngest most vulnerable. The focus of India's current nutrition programmes has become supplementary nutrition and pre-school education for four to six year olds, belying the need to focus adequately on the first two years of a child's life—critical to prevent undernutrition and its sequelae. Even breastfeeding should be advocated as a universal practice up to at least 6 months of the infant's age, the circumstances that govern the life of a poor working mother (who has access to neither maternity leave nor a nearby crèche) must be borne in mind. In urban areas, the decline in food insecurity between 2000 and 2006 has been by a margin of only 0.4 per cent, out of step with the 6 per cent growth rate in the same period. Nutrition is a social determinant of health and is itself influenced by many other social determinants. Vertical programmes will, therefore, not provide complete or lasting solutions.

(b) Water and Sanitation

There is a clear correlation between inadequate and poor quality of water or sanitation and health. A study of urban poor communities in Mumbai found that water-related illnesses accounted for almost a third of all morbidity in the last year among adults, and almost two-thirds of all morbidity among children. Another study in five Indian states found a negative correlation between the provision of household toilets and community-level prevalence of communicable diseases including cholera, typhoid/enteric disease, diarrhoea/vomiting, hepatitis, and nematodal infections as well as malaria and dengue. A 2002 Planning Commission report expressed alarm over the 'rather extensive presence' of fluoride and arsenic in Indian drinking water, which is associated with a number of cancers (of the skin, lungs, kidneys, and bladder). According to the Water and Sanitation Programme, the cost per Disability Adjusted Life Year (DALY) of poor sanitation in urban areas is estimated at 5,400 INR. Another major finding is that use of improved facilities is strongly correlated with sanitation-related knowledge and hygiene-promotive attitudes.

(c) Social Exclusion

In rural India, women are three times more likely than men to go without treatment for long-term ailments, a trend that persists even among the non-poor. When treatment is sought, significantly smaller sums of money are spent on treatment of women than on men. Provisional data from the 2011 Census suggests that gender inequity is a persistent and worsening phenomenon in India, occurring throughout the life cycle: a 13-point decline in the male-female sex ratio from 927 females per 1,000 males in 2001 to 914 females per 1,000 males in 2011 suggests that as more families are having fewer children, gendering of sex composition is rising. Girls that survive till adolescence must navigate situations of both wanton neglect and unwanted attention: a study of backward districts in 12 Indian states found that 88 per cent of adolescent girls were undernourished while almost two-thirds (64.6%) reported some form of sexual abuse.

Apart from gender, social status is also associated with systemic neglect and poor health. Caste and social stratification in India determines health, education, employment, social, and economic outcomes. For example, Indians in the lowest socio-economic stratum presently experience cardiovascular disease in greater proportions than those in higher strata. National Sample Survey Data (NSSD) reveals that by controlling a number of determinants (such as gender, residence in a forward or backward state, urban or rural area, living conditions, and socio-economic status), the mean age of death was 5–7 years lower among STs and SCs and 6–9 years lower among Muslims in comparison to Hindus.

The HLEG (2011) report also finds that in Kerala, a state with good health outcomes, the odds of reporting poor health are 88 per cent higher among ST/SC and 73 per cent higher among OBC women as compared to forward castes (in 2006). The gravity of caste-based social exclusion is seeing recognition in the incorporation of this indicator in the 2011 Census. The health of tribal populations is also of particular concern. The latest National Family Health Survey (NFHS–3) found a complete lack of treatment for diarrhoea for over a third of respondents from scheduled tribes (36.3%), as compared to 27.6 per cent among scheduled castes (SCs), 28.2 per cent among other backward castes (OBCs), and less than a quarter among the rest of the Indian population (23.8%). Multiple studies have found that tribal children face the greatest incidence of malnutrition in India, particularly in the states of Jharkhand, Bihar, Madhya Pradesh, Chhattisgarh, Odisha, and West Bengal. There are significant inter-state differences in health. The infant mortality rate in the state of Kerala is 17 deaths per 1,000 live births as compared to 111 deaths per 1,000 live births in Madhya Pradesh.

According to the 2011 Census, while Punjab's child sex ratio improved from 798 females per 1,000 males in 2001 to 846 females per 1,000 males in 2011, this figure still remains among the lowest in India. Moreover, while maternal mortality declined by 32.4 per cent between 2001–03 and 2004–06 in West Bengal, Haryana registered a 3 per cent increase in the same period.

(d) Work (In)Security, Occupational Health, and Disasters

Globalization and the concomitant casualization of labour have resulted in the growth of informal economies that account for 93 per cent of the Indian workforce. Migrant workers are among the poorest and most exploited, performing low level, unskilled, and hazardous work. This population faces significant disease burdens including musculoskeletal injuries, chronic obstructive lung diseases, toxic chemical exposure and poisoning, and noise-induced hearing loss. Rapid urbanization has spurred concentration of services and industries in cities, at times making them epicentres of protracted public health disasters, like the 1984 methyl-isocyanate leak in Bhopal. In rare cases, like the plague in Surat, social determinants of health crises have catalysed reforms in sanitation and health services. Civil conflict is also associated with poor health: political combatants and refugees in Chhattisgarh face syndemics of malnutrition, malaria, and other communicable diseases.

References

Advani, M. and Akram, M. (2007). 'Health Concerns in India', in M. Akram (ed.), *Health Dynamics and Marginalised Communities* (pp. 3–26), Jaipur: Rawat Publications.

Akram, M. (2012b). 'Development of Sociology of Health: A Review of the Contexts and Phases, Themes and Future in India', *Salute e Società, (Sociology and Sociology of Health: A Round Trip)*, XI-2 (English), 89–115.

Calnan, M. (1987). *Health and Illness: The Lay Perspective*, London: Tavistock Publications.

Dingwall, R. (1976). *Aspects of Illness*, London: Martin Robertson

Giddens, A. (2006). *Sociology*, fifth edition, Cambridge: Polity Press.

HLEG. (2011). Available online at: http://planningcommission.nic.in/reports/genrep/rep_uhc0812.pdf. (accessed 6 July 2012).

Hobson, W. (ed.). (1965). *The Theory and Practice of Public Health*, New York: Oxford University Press.

Kelman, S. (1975). 'The Social Nature of the Definition Problem in Health', *International Journal of Health Services*, 5: 625–642.

Kleinman, A. (1988). *The Illness Narratives: Suffering, Healing and the Human Condition*, New York: Basic Books.

McKenzie, J.F., Pinger, R.R. and Kotecki, J.E. (2002). *An Introduction to Community Health*, fourth edition, Massachusetts: Jones and Bartlett Publishers.

Nettleton, S. (1995). *The Sociology of Health and Illness*, UK: Polity Press.

Park, K. (2005). *Preventive and Social Medicine* 18th edition, Jabalpur: Banarsidas Bhanot.

WHO. (2005). Resolution WHA58.33. 'Sustainable Health Financing, Universal Coverage and Social Health Insurance', in *Fifty-eighth World Health Assembly*, 16–25 May 2005. Geneva, WHO, 2005. Available online at: http://apps.who.int/gb/ebwha/pdf_files/WHA58/WHA58_33–en.pdf (accessed 23 June 2010).

WHO. (2010). *The World Health Report: Health Systems Financing: The Path to Universal Coverage*. Available online at: www.who.int/entity/whr/2010/overview.pdf (accessed 5 July 2012).

Chapter Ten

Health Indicators in India

Indicators help to measure the extent to which the objectives and targets of a programme are being attained. A health indicator is a variable—that can be measured directly to reflect the state of health of people within a community. Health indicators are required not only to measure the health status of a community but also to compare the health status of country with that of other; for assessment of health care needs; for allocation of health care resources; and for monitoring and evaluation of health services, activities, and programmes. In WHO guidelines for health programme evaluation, health indicators are defined as variables that help to measure changes. Park (2009), in his book *Preventive and Social Medicine,* mentions good number of indicators of health. Some of the important indicators of health, also discussed by Park, are presented here in this chapter.

Mortality Indicators

Mortality refers to the death process characterizing a population. The study of mortality examines the relationship between death and the size, composition, and distribution of the population. Furthermore, mortality studies investigate the 'who, how, why, and when' issues related to dying. Medical sociologists have contributed greatly to the understanding of the factors contributing to mortality and the distribution of mortality within the population (Thomas, 2002). The study of mortality is an important area of social epidemiology, particularly in societies that are less developed and are affected more by acute conditions than chronic conditions. Mortality like fertility is significantly influenced by socio-cultural factors and even age-specific deaths are to a certain extent a function of non-biological factors. These include characteristics such as marital status and family structure, socio-economic status, occupation, industry and employment status, lifestyle, and even religion. Mortality rates include following:

(a) Expectation of Life

Expectation of life refers to average expected life of an individual at the time of his birth. When expected life of an individual is long, it reflects good state of health and control over morbidity conditions and vice versa. It is estimated for both sexes separately. For the period of 1996–2001, the life expectancy at birth is estimated to be 62.36 years for males and 63 years for females. As an indicator of long-term survival, it can be considered as a positive health indicator. The increased life expectancy and uneven performance between fertility and mortality rates have posed dual challenges to simultaneously improve both primary and secondary health care services. The life expectancy at birth has increased to 59.7 for male and 60.9 years for female in 1991–95 from 58.1 and 58.6 years for male and female respectively during 1987–91. The technical group on population, Registrar General of India, has projected levels of expectation of life during 2001–06 as 63.87 years for male and 66.97 for female, demanding specialized health care services for the increased number of older persons (India, National Health System Profile: 04).

Life expectancy in India has more than doubled in the last 60 years. It increased from around 30 years at the time of independence to over 63.5 years in 2002–06. Although the decadal increase has slowed from 5.7 years in the 1970s to 3.2 years in the 1990s, the overall life expectancy is increased by 14.1 years in the rural areas and 9.9 years in the urban areas during the period

1970–75 to 2002–06. The wide variance in performance across states is of special concern. While in Kerala, a person at the time of birth is expected to live for 74 years, the expectancy of life at birth in states such as Assam, Bihar, Madhya Pradesh, Orissa, Rajasthan, and Uttar Pradesh is in the range of 58–62 years, a level Kerala achieved during the period 1970–75. Globally India's life expectancy is lower than the global average of 67.5 years and the average of most countries that won their independence from colonial rule at about the same time—China, Vietnam, Sri Lanka, and so on (Annual Report to the People on Health, September 2010, Government of India, Ministry of Health and Family Welfare). Life expectancy at birth for the whole population across 22 Asian countries reached 71.6 years on average in 2008, and the country with the longest life expectancy in 2008 was Japan, with a combined value for men and women of 82.7 years (OECD, 2010).

(b) Crude Death Rate (CDR)

The Crude Death Rate (CDR) expresses deaths as the number per 1,000 populations. It is defined as the number of deaths per 1,000 population per year in a given community. It indicates the rate at which people are dying. Reducing the number of deaths in the population is an obvious goal of medicine and health care and success or failure to do so is a measure of a nation's commitment to better health.

(c) Total Fertility Rate (TFR)

Total Fertility Rate (TFR) is the average number of children that a woman would bear over her lifetime if she were to experience the current age-specific fertility rates. At a level of 2.1, which is called the replacement level, population stabilization could be said to have been achieved. TFR of India had reduced from 5.2 in 1971 to 2.6 in 2008. Of concern are the states of Uttar Pradesh, Bihar, Jharkhand, Rajasthan, Madhya Pradesh, and Chhattisgarh that account for over 40 per cent of India's population and have a TFR in the range of 3.0 to 3.9—a level that Kerala and Tamil Nadu had in the early 1970s. India's record compares poorly with that of Japan, China, and the United Sates, which have TFRs of 1.3, 1.7, and 2.1, respectively. As per population projections, the population of India in the year 2025 will be 143.1 crore as compared to 145.3 crore of China. TFR varies significantly with female literacy, mean age of women at marriage, percentage of females working in non-primary sectors, infant and child mortality, type of housing, and level of urbanization. The TFR declines significantly with the level of education of the mother. Scheduled tribes have the highest level of TFR followed by scheduled castes, other backward classes, and others.

(d) Child and Infant Mortality Rate

Child Mortality Rate is defined as the number of deaths at ages 1–4 years in a given year, per 1,000 children in that age group. Child mortality is usually measured using three indicators: Neonatal Mortality Rate (NMR—less than 1 month), Infant Mortality Rate (IMR—less than 1 year), and Under-5 Mortality Rate (U5MR). Table 1 lists the states and union territories in India, which have a

Table 1 States with high neonatal mortality rate (NMR), IMR, and under-5 mortality rates

Name of the State	*NMR (SRS 2006)*	*IMR (SRS 2007)*	*U5 MR (NFHS–3, 2005)*
Madhya Pradesh	51	74	94
Orissa	52	73	90
Uttar Pradesh	46	71	96
Assam	35	67	85
Rajasthan	45	67	85
Chhattisgarh	43	61	90
Bihar	32	60	84
Haryana	34	57	52
Andhra Pradesh	33	56	63
Gujarat	38	53	60
Meghalaya	NA	53	70
Jammu and Kashmir	39	52	51
Himachal Pradesh	30	50	41
Jharkhand	29	49	93
Karnataka	28	48	54
Punjab	30	44	52
Uttarakhand	NA	43	56
Arunachal Pradesh	NA	40	87

Source: Ramani, Mavalankar, Joshi, Malek, Puvar, and Kumar, (April–June 2010): 9–10 and Sample Registration System (SRS).

very high neonatal, infant, and U5 mortality rates. India is a large and diverse country with wide variations across the states on NMR, IMR, and U5MR. On the one hand, we have states like Kerala and Tamil Nadu having excellent indicators of child health, comparable with those of many developed countries. On the other hand, we have states like Orissa, Madhya Pradesh, UP, Rajasthan, and Bihar, whose child health indicators are very poor. These five states put together account for almost 40 per cent of India's total population and 60 per cent of the child deaths.

Globally, more than 10 million children under 5 years of age, almost all in poor countries die every year (20 children per minute), mostly from preventable causes. A few countries account for a large proportion of child deaths and India tops this list. In the year 2000, eight countries in the world accounted for 60 per cent of all child deaths. While 42 countries accounted for 90 per cent of the child deaths (Black, Morris and Bryce, 2003), forty per cent of the child deaths occurred in the four Asian countries, namely, India, China, Pakistan, and Bangladesh.

(e) Infant Mortality Rate (IMR)

The infant mortality rate is one of the important statistics for measuring the health of a population. It is defined as the number of children who die before reaching their first birthday in a given year, expressed per 1,000 live births. It is a sensitive indicator of the availability, utilization, and effectiveness of the health care, particularly perinatal care. India's infant mortality rate too has shown a steady decline, from 77 deaths per 1,000 live births in 1991–95 (10–14 years before the survey) to 57 deaths per 1,000 live births in 2001–05 (0–4 years before the survey), thus implying an average rate of decline of 2 infant deaths per 1,000 live births per year (MoHFW, 2010; NFHS–3, 2007: 179).

Infant and child mortality rates are considerably higher in rural areas than in urban areas. In 2001–05, the infant mortality rate was 50 per cent higher in rural areas (62) than in urban areas (42). The rural-urban difference in mortality is especially large for children in the age interval 1–4 years, while the rate in rural areas is twice as high as the rate in urban areas. In both the neonatal and postneonatal periods, mortality in rural areas is about 50 per cent higher than mortality in urban areas. Infant and child mortality rates have declined slightly faster in rural areas than in urban areas. Between 1991–95 and 2001–05, infant mortality declined by 27 per cent in rural areas, compared with 21 per cent in urban areas. During the same period, the child mortality rate declined by 45 per cent in rural areas, compared with 40 per cent in urban areas. Even in the neonatal period, the decline in mortality was slightly faster in rural areas (26%) than in urban areas (18%).

(f) Under-five Mortality Rates

There have been considerable efforts to reduce under-five mortality rates in the country over the last three decades. In 2002, the average under-five mortality rate in India was 85 deaths per 1,000 live births, a considerable reduction as compared to 202 in 1970. The rate of decline in the 1990s, however, is about half of previous decade's rate of decline 4.7 per cent. At the current rate, India would achieve under-five mortality of 64 per 1,000 live births by 2015, which is well short of Millennium Development Goal (MDG) of 41.

(g) Maternal Mortality

Maternal mortality in India continues to be a major concern given the reduced social, cultural, and economic status of Indian women that inhibits them from adequate access to health facilities. Maternal mortality is defined as the death of a woman during pregnancy or childbirth or in the 42 days after delivery from any cause that is related to or aggravated by the pregnancy (OECD, 2010). Maternal mortality is measured using the Maternal Mortality Ratio (MMR), that is, the number of maternal deaths in a population divided by the number of live births in a given year. MMR assesses the risk of maternal death relative to the number of live births. It is higher in the countries where the women are illiterate and orthodox; where the death of the women is not very cared for; less gap between children; and where child marriages prevail. India had an MMR of 460 in 1984, declining to 254 deaths per 1,00,000 live births in 2004–06. The level of maternal mortality varies greatly by state, with Kerala and Tamil Nadu reporting MMR of 95 and 111 per lakh respectively, lower than Assam (480),

Bihar/Jharkhand (312), Madhya Pradesh/Chhattisgarh (335), Orissa (303), Rajasthan (388), and Uttar Pradesh/Uttarakhand (440). This is most likely related to differences in the socio-economic status of women and access to health care services among the states (MoHFW, 2010).

There are several causes attributed to maternal deaths. Some of the direct causes, such as haemorrhage, puerperal complications, obstructed labour, abortions, and toxaemia, account for more than three-fourths of the maternal deaths, while other related causes such as anaemia, pregnancy with TB/malaria, viral hepatitis, and others account for rest of the deaths (Raj, 2007). Studies have shown that haemorrhage, sepsis, and anaemia are the major causes of maternal deaths, more so in rural areas. NFHS–2 reveals that moderate and severe anaemia among pregnant women (28%) is almost double than that of non-pregnant women (16%). Apart from these, there are several other intangible factors associated with maternal deaths. They are overall health status, reproductive status, access to health services, and extent of utilization of health services. Adoption or non-adoption of family planning service also in a way has an effect on maternal mortality. The high maternal death rate is further reflected with the performance of pregnancy-related indicators. According to NFHS–3, only 51 per cent of mothers received antenatal check-up (at least three visits), 71 per cent received two or more doses of tetanus toxoid, and contraceptive prevalence is 56.3 per cent in 2005–06 (India, National Health System Profile).

(h) Disease-Specific Mortality

Mortality rates can be computed for specific diseases. As countries begin to extricate themselves from the burden of communicable diseases, a number of other indicators such as deaths from cancer, cardiovascular diseases, accidents diabetes, etc., have emerged as measures of specific disease problems.

Morbidity Indicators

The study of morbidity is perhaps the most important dimension of social epidemiology, particularly in modern industrialized societies. Historically, morbidity, or the level of sickness and disability within a population, has been an area of study for both clinicians and population-oriented scientists such as epidemiologists. In recent years, however, increased activity on the part of social scientists has been observed, as researchers apply various methodologies and perspectives to the study of sickness and disability (Thomas, 2002). The health status of a population is reflected in the levels of morbidity and the treatment seeking behaviours of its members. For Advani and Akram (2007), mortality rate alone is not a good indicator of health of a society because death after certain age is also natural. Mortality rate does not reveal the burden of ill health in a community. On the other hand, it is the morbidity that reflects the number of persons affected with some disease and hence indicates ill health. Therefore, morbidity indicators are used to supplement mortality data to describe the health status of a population. The morbidity rates, which are used for assessing ill health in the community, are: (a) incidence and prevalence, (b) notification rates, (c) duration of stay in hospitals, and (d) spells of sickness or absence from work or school (Park, 2009).

The NFHS–3 (2007) informs about four major diseases prevailing in India (asthma, tuberculosis, jaundice, malaria): 1,600 persons per 1,00,000 populations in India were reported to be suffering from asthma at the time of survey. Asthma is a chronic respiratory disease characterized by sudden attacks of laboured breathing, chest constriction, and coughing. There has been a rapid increase in asthma cases in recent years in many parts of the world. In India, the prevalence of asthma is high in rural areas than in urban areas and is slightly higher in males than in females (1,719 per 1,00,000 for women and 1,799 per 1,00,000 for men). The highest levels of asthma are seen among less educated persons. Prevalence is highest among those with less than five years of schooling (2,283 among women and 2,640 among men), and among those with no education (1,914 among women and 2,440 among men).

Tuberculosis (TB), which is also resurgent worldwide, is an infectious disease that affects the lungs and other body tissues. Tuberculosis of the lungs, the most commonly known form, is characterized by coughing up mucus and sputum, fever, weight loss, and chest pain. The overall prevalence of tuberculosis in India is 445 per 1,00,000 populations. The risk of TB is much higher for men (526/1,00,000) than women (309/1,00,000) because males are in contact with more people who might have TB and smoking is more in men, and much higher for rural residents (469/100,000) than urban residents (307/1,00,000). TB prevalence increases with increasing age. Persons age 60 and above (998/1,00,000) are much more likely than other age groups to be suffering from tuberculosis. Prevalence in the oldest age group is about twice as high as prevalence in the population age 15–59 (519/100,000) and about nine times as high as prevalence among children below age 15 (110/1,00,000). Both sex and age differentials are more pronounced in rural areas than they are in urban areas.

Jaundice is characterized by yellowish discolouration of the eyes and skin, fever, liver enlargement, and abdominal pain. Jaundice cases were reported to be 1361 persons per 100,000 populations. This is more prevalent in rural areas than in urban areas. However, it decreases with age. Thus, highest numbers of jaundice patients are in the age of 0–14.

Malaria is characterized by recurrent high fever with shivering. The overall prevalence of malaria in India is 3,697 persons per 1,00,000 populations. People of rural area suffer twice than that of urban area and it is slightly high for males than for females. All these diseases, however, vary and differ from state to state depending on the climate and geographical locations of the areas.

Nutritional Status Indicators

Nutritional adequacy is one of the positive key determinants of health and well-being of the children. Over half (54%) of all childhood deaths in India are related to malnutrition (Bajpai and Dholakia, 2011). Globally, maternal and child under nutrition is the underlying cause of 3.5 million deaths every year, 35 per cent of the disease burden in children under 5, and 11 per cent total days lost. Undernutrition occurs due to protein and energy malnutrition as well as micronutrient deficiency. In 2005–06, about 44 per cent of Indian children under 5 were underweight, and 48 per cent were stunted due to chronic malnutrition. Due to the country's size, this means that India is home to 42 per cent of the world's underweight children and 31 per cent of the world's stunted children.

The proportion of stunted and undernourished children in India is 19–21 times higher than expected for a healthy, well-nourished population according to international child growth standards. High levels of child undernutrition are driven by the low nutritional and social status of women. Forty per cent of women in India have low body mass, a factor in low birth-weight. Twenty-eight per cent of children born in India are low birth-weight, indicating intrauterine undernutrition. Nearly half of low-birth-weight babies are currently stunted or underweight, compared to one-third of normal birth-weight babies (NFHS–3). Nearly 40 per cent of all low-birth-weight babies in the world are born in India (Bajpai and Dholakia, 2011). Undernourishment in children retards physical development and hampers the learning and cognitive processes leading to sluggish educational, social, and economic development. Ignoring undernutrition puts the long-term health and development of population at risk. Park (2009) mentions that anthropometric measurements of preschool children, for example, weight, height, mid-arm circumference; height of children at school entry; prevalence of low birth weight (less than 2.5 kg), etc., constitute nutritional status indicators.

Adequate nutrition is critical to child development. The period from birth to two years of age is important for optimal growth, health, and development. At this age, children are particularly vulnerable to growth retardation, micronutrient deficiencies, and common childhood illnesses such as diarrhoea and acute respiratory infections (ARI). Malnutrition in women and men can result in reduced productivity, slow recovery from illnesses, increased susceptibility to infections, and a heightened risk of adverse pregnancy outcomes. A woman's nutritional status has important implications for her health as well as the health of her children. A woman with poor nutritional status, as indicated by a low body mass index (BMI), short stature, anaemia, or other micronutrient deficiencies, has a greater risk of obstructed labour, having a baby with a low-birth weight, having adverse pregnancy outcomes, producing lower quality breast milk, death due to postpartum haemorrhage, and illness for herself and her baby (NFHS–3, 2007).

Earlier it has been noted that various studies indicate that malnutrition is one of the serious health problem for Indian women. It threatens their survival as well as that of their children. The negative effects of malnutrition in women are compounded by heavy work demands, poverty, childbearing and rearing, and the special nutritional needs of women, resulting in increased susceptibility to illness and consequent higher mortality. While malnutrition in India is prevalent among all segments of the population, poor nutrition among women begins in infancy and continues throughout their lifetimes. Women and girls are typically the last to eat in a family; thus, if there is not enough food they are the ones who suffer most.

Three standard indices of physical growth that describe the nutritional status of children are as follows:

- Height-for-age (stunting)
- Weight-for-height (wasting)
- Weight-for-age (underweight)

Table 2 Nutritional status of children and the ever-married women

Feeding practice/nutritional status (%)	*Data source*		
	NFHS (1992–93)	*NFHS (1998–99)*	*NFHS (2005–06)*
Children			
<3 years breastfed within 1 hour of birth	9.5	16	23.4
0–5 months exclusively breastfed	0	0	46.3
6–9 months receiving solid or semi-solid food and breast milk	0	0	55.8
<3 years who are stunted	0	45.5	38.4
< 3 years who are wasted	0	15.5	19.1
< 3 years who are underweight	51.5	47	45.9
Ever-married women 15–49 years			
Body mass index < normal	0	36.2	33
Overweight or obese	0	10.6	14.8

Source: Saha and Saha (2010).

An unhealthy mother gives birth to an unhealthy child. As per the data given in Table 2, Indian children have among the highest incidence of malnourishment in the world. More than half (53%) of all girls and boys under four years were malnourished, and a similar proportion (52%) was stunted (too short for their age). Other studies show that many women never achieve full physical development. This incomplete physical development poses the considerable risk for women of obstructed obstetric deliveries.

'The mother's education is highly correlated with the level of malnutrition among children. The children of illiterate mothers are twice as likely to be undernourished or stunted as are children whose mothers have completed at least high school. The differentials are even larger when severely undernourished children are considered. Children of illiterate mothers are three times as likely to be severely undernourished as children of mothers with at least a high school education. The nutritional status of children also differs by state. Bihar and Uttar Pradesh have the highest proportion of undernourished children and Kerala has the lowest, consistent with the different levels of socio-economic development in these states. However, NFHS–3 reports that the proportion of children under 3 years who are underweight decreased from 18 per cent to 16 per cent. Stunting decreased by a larger margin, from 51 per cent to 45 per cent. Severe stunting also decreased from 28 per cent to 22 per cent. The decrease of stunting over time was greater in rural areas than urban areas but the prevalence of children who were underweight decreased slight more in urban areas than in rural areas' (Saha and Saha, 2010: 7).

Maternal Health Indicators

Maternal health is a key indicator of women's health and status. Maternal health refers to the health of women during pregnancy, childbirth, and the postpartum period. Pregnancy and childbirth are of course not diseases. But, they carry risks because of the varying and embedded complications, practices, processes, beliefs, life conditions, and the immediate environment. These risks can be reduced by health care interventions such as the provision of maternal and public health care, supplementary nutrition, family planning, safe abortion, and improvement in other reproductive conditions.

(a) Antenatal Care

According to NFHS–3, antenatal care (ANC) refers to pregnancy-related health care, which is usually provided by a doctor, an ANM, or another health professional. Ideally, antenatal care should monitor a pregnancy for signs of complications, detect and treat pre-existing and concurrent problems of pregnancy, and provide advice and counselling on preventive care, diet during pregnancy, delivery care, postnatal care, and related issues. The most commonly reported pregnancy-related health problems are excessive fatigue (48%) and swelling of the legs, body, or face (25%). Ten per cent of mothers had convulsions that were not from fever and 9 per cent reported night blindness.

(b) Assistance during Delivery

Forty-seven per cent of births in the five years preceding the survey (NFHS–3) were assisted by health personnel, including 35 per cent by a doctor and 10 per cent by an ANM, nurse, midwife, or LHV. More than one-third of births (37%) were assisted by a traditional birth attendant (TBA) and 16 per cent were assisted by only friends, relatives, or other persons. Based on mothers' reports, 9 per cent of children born in India in the 5 years before the survey were delivered by caesarean section. The proportion of deliveries by caesarean section was three times as high in urban areas (17%) as in rural areas (6%). Twenty-eight per cent of births delivered in private health facilities and 15 per cent of births delivered in public sector health facilities were delivered by caesarean section.

(c) Overall Care

For India as a whole, mothers of only 15 per cent of births received all of the required components of antenatal care. This indicator ranges from a high of 64 per cent in Kerala and 56 per cent in Goa to a low of only 2 per cent in Nagaland and 4 per cent in Uttar Pradesh. Other states that performed almost as poorly as Uttar Pradesh and Nagaland on this indicator included Bihar, Arunachal Pradesh, Madhya Pradesh, Jharkhand, Meghalaya, Rajasthan, and Mizoram, where only 6–9 per cent of women received the recommended components of antenatal care.

Health Care Delivery Indicators

The frequently used health care delivery indicators are: (a) doctor-population ratio, (b) doctor-nurse ratio, (c) population bed ratio, (d) population per health centre, and (e) population per traditional birth attendant. These indicators reflect the equity of distribution of health resources in different parts of the country and of the provision of health care (Park, 2009). Institutional delivery is one such indicator. Less than 40 per cent of births in India took place in health facilities. More than half took place in the woman's own home, and 9 per cent took place in the parents' home. Births in health facilities were equally divided between those that took place in a private health facility and those that took place in public institutions (such as government-operated district, tehsil/taluk, town, or municipal hospitals, and Primary Health Centres). Two-thirds of deliveries in urban areas and 29 per cent of deliveries in rural areas took place in health facilities (NFHS–3, 2007).

Indicators of Social and Mental Health

Mental health refers to people's cognitive and emotional well-being. A person who enjoys good mental health does not have a mental disorder. WHO defines mental health as 'the capacity of the individual, the group, and the environment to interact with one another in ways that promote subjective well-being, the optimal development and use of mental abilities (cognitive, affective, and relational), the achievement of individual and collective goals consistent with justice, and the attainment and preservation of conditions of fundamental equality' (Gangolli, Duggal, and Shukla, 2005: 127). 'This definition not only keeps the individual at the centre but also goes beyond in connecting it with the larger social context. Suicide, homicide, acts of violence, crime, road traffic accidents, juvenile delinquency, alcohol and drug abuse, smoking, obesity, battered baby, battered wife syndromes, etc., constitute the social and mental health indicators. These social indicators provide a guide to social action for improving the health of people' (Park, 2009: 26).

'Social and mental or psychological circumstances can cause long-term stress. Continuing anxiety, insecurity, low self-esteem, social isolation, and control over work and home life have powerful effects on health. Such psychosocial risks accumulate during life and increase the chances of poor mental health and premature death. Long periods of anxiety and insecurity and the lack of supportive friendships are damaging in whatever area of life they arise. The lower the people's position in social hierarchy of industrialized countries, the more common these problems become' (Wilkinson and Mormot, 2003: 12).

Socio-economic Indicators

These include: (a) rate of population increase, (b) per capita GNP, (c) level of unemployment, (d) family size and literacy rates-especially female literacy rates, housing and also per-capita 'calorie' availability. These indicators do not directly measure health. Nevertheless they have great importance in the interpretation of the indicators of health care. Social indicators as defined by the United Nations Statistical office (UNSO), have been divided into twelve categories: population, family formation, families and households, learning and education services, learning accumulation, social security and welfare services, health services and nutrition, housing and its environment, leisure and culture, social stratification and morbidity.

Health Policy Indicator

Park (2009) mentions that the single most important indicator of political commitment is 'allocation of adequate resources'. The relevant indicators are: (i) proportion of GNP spent on health services, (ii) proportion of GNP spent on health-related activities (water supply, sanitation, housing, and nutrition), and (iii) proportion of total health resources devoted to primary health care.

Environmental Indicators

Environmental indicators reflect the quality of social, physical, and biological environment in which diseases occur and in which people live. They include indicators relating to pollution of air, water, radiations, solid wastes, noise, exposure of toxic substances in food or drink, and stress. Among these the most useful indicators are those measuring the proportion of population having access to safe water and sanitation facilities. Contaminated water and poor sanitation is responsible for large proportion of diseases in India. Poor hygiene and sanitation account for 9 per cent of all deaths is estimated each year in India (for details, see Akram, 2012).

Utilization Rates

In order to get more information on health status, the extent of use of health services is often investigated. Utilization of services or actual coverage is expressed as the proportion of people in need of a service who actually receive it in a given period, usually a year. Utilization rates give some indication of the care needed by a population and therefore the health status of a population. For example, (i) proportion of infants who are fully immunized, (ii) bed occupancy rate (i.e., average daily in-patient/average number of beds), (iii) average length of staying in a hospital, and (iv) bed turnover ratio, etc.

Besides these health indicators, the other health indicators are quality of life, basic health indicators, health for all indicators, millennium development goal indicators, etc. The search for indicators associated with or casually related to health continues. Thus, it can be seen from the above that there is no single comprehensive indicator of a nation's health and each available indicators reflect an aspect of health.

References

Akram, M. (2012). 'Challenges Before Health Planning in India: Preparing Draft of the 12th Five-year Plan', *Journal of US-China Public Administration*, 9(2): 229–234.

Bajpai, N. and Dholakia, R.H. (2011). *Improving the Integration of Health and Nutrition Sectors in India*, Columbia Global Centres/South Asia, Columbia University.

Black, R.E., Morris, S.S. and Bryce, J. (2003). 'Where and why are 10 million children dying every year?', *Lancet*, 361: 2226–34

Gangolli, L.V., Duggal, R. and Shukla, A. (2005). *Review of Healthcare in India*, Mumbai: Centre for Enquiry into Health and Allied Themes, Research Centre of Anusandhan Trust, Survey No. 2804 and 2805.

India, National Health System Profile, (year not mentioned) PDF, p. 04,. Available online at: 209.61.208.233/LinkFiles/India_CHP_india.pdf (accessed on 10 June 2012).

MoHFW. (September 2010). *Annual Report to the People on Health*, Government of India, Ministry of Health and Family Welfare, Nirman Bhawan, New Delhi.

NFHS–3, 2005–06, India, Vol. I, September 2007, International Institute for Population Sciences, Govandi Station Road, Deonar, Mumbai.

OECD. (2010). *Health at a Glance: Asia/Pacific 2010*, OECD Publishing. Available online at: http://dx.doi.org/10.1787/9789264096202–en. (accessed on 18 May 2012).

Park, K. (2009). *Preventive and Social Medicine* 20th edition, Jabalpur: Banarsidas Bhanot.

Raj, H. (2007). *Fundamentals of Demography*, New Delhi: Surjeet Publications.

Ramani, K.V., Mavalankar, D., Joshi, S., Malek, I., Puvar, T. and Kumar, H. (2010). 'Why Should 5,000 Children Die in India Every Day? Major Causes of Death and Managerial Challenges', *Vikalpa*, volume 35(2).

Saha, U.C. and Saha, K.B. (2010). 'A Trend in Women's Health in India—What Has Been Achieved and What Can Be Done', *Rural and Remote Health*. Available online at: http://www.rrh.org.au. (accessed on 10 May 2012).

Thomas, R.K. (2002). *Society and Health: Sociology for Health Professionals*, New York: Kluwer Academic Publishers.

Wilkinson, R. and Mormot, M. (2003). *Social Determinants of Health: The Solid Facts*, second edition, International Centre for Health and Society. WHO available at: http://www.euro.who.int/__data/assets/pdf_file/0005/98438/e81384.pdf (accessed on 21 April 2012).

www.jeywin.com

http://dx.doi.org/10.1787/9789264096202–en

http://www.medicalnewstoday.com/articles/150999.php

CHAPTER ELEVEN

Occupational Health

The joint ILO/WHO committee on occupational health, in its first session, held in 1950, defined occupational health by explaining its aims: 'occupational health should aim at the promotion and maintenance of the highest degree of physical, mental and social well-being of workers in all occupations; the prevention amongst workers of departures from health caused by their working conditions; the protection of workers in their employment from risks resulting from factors adverse to health; the placing and maintenance of the worker in an occupational environment adapted to his physiological and psychological capabilities and; to summarize: the adaptation of work to man and of each man to his job'. Cherilyn Tillman (2007) has defined occupational health as the maintenance of the individual worker's state of well-being and freedom from occupationally related disease or injury. According to Park, 'the goal of the preventive medicine and occupational health is the same—that is, prevention of disease and maintenance of the highest degree of physical, mental, and social well-being of workers in all occupations; specific protection of workers; early diagnosis and treatment; disability limitation and rehabilitation, etc. Therefore, occupational health is the application of preventive medicine in all places of employment' (2009: 708).

Park further says, 'it was customary in the past to think of occupational health entirely in relation to factories and mines: hence, the terms 'industrial health' or 'industrial hygiene' were in vogue. Modern concepts of occupational health now include all types of employment including mercantile and commercial enterprises, service trades, forestry and agriculture, and include the subjects of industrial hygiene, industrial diseases, industrial accidents, industrial hazards, industrial rehabilitation, and occupational psychology. Occupational health in agriculture and ergonomics (human engineering) are relatively new concepts' (ibid.: 708).

Kevin White (2006) notes that our occupation exposes us to a wide range of physical and psychosocial risks. These range from high-risk industries in which occupation can be easily shown to be the sole cause of cancer, as in the asbestos industry. Overall it is estimated that 20 per cent of all cancer deaths can be attributed to occupation. The stress of work environments that combine low autonomy and high workloads in an unsupportive environment has been claimed to be the cause of up to 35 per cent of cardiovascular mortality. In Australia, an estimated 500 workers die each year at work, a further 2,200 die of work-related cancers and 6,50,000 are injured or become sick directly because of their work.

Globally, there are more than 2.6 billion workers and the workforce is growing continuously. Approximately, 75 per cent of these workers are in developing countries where workplace hazards are more severe. Each year there are as many as 250 million occupational injuries resulting in 3,30,000 fatalities. Each day in the United States, on average 15 workers die from an injury sustained at work. If one includes occupational illnesses, an estimated 1.1 million people worldwide die each year. Annually, an estimated 160 million new cases of work-related diseases occur worldwide. All of these estimates are almost certainly below the actual figures because the reports from many areas of the world are unreliable (McKenzie, Pinger, and Kotecki, 2005).

According to Tillman (2007), society does not expect workers to trade away their health and safety just to have a job. But occupationally related illness can still occur in many workplaces and not just in industrial workplaces. Chemicals, which are potentially capable of causing cancer, lung diseases, blood and bone disorders, loss of mental ability, central nervous system debilitation, infertility, and death, are still found in factories and farms. Microbiological hazards coexist with humans and contribute to poor indoor air quality or present significant risk of infectious diseases in animal handling, childcare, nursing and hospital care, or community services where accidental body fluid exchange can occur. Industrial workplaces can also put physical and mental strains on the worker—for example, manual handling, noise, vibration, extremes of heat and cold, and exposure to both ionizing and non-ionizing radiation. Humans have no natural protection against extreme exposures to any of these. All of these hazards contribute to make many workplaces potentially unhealthy.

Occupational health is a multidimensional field encompassing science, social progress, economics, law, employment studies, and issues common to every family. The health and safety of people at work is a critical concern for all societies and all countries. The field of occupational health touches on fundamental aspects of working life:

- making a living
- providing for a family
- staying healthy
- avoiding unnecessary risk of injury
- protecting oneself and others from harm
- creating useful products and services for societal benefit
- anticipating and preventing future problems
- sharing information
- the right to knowledge of potential health hazards
- fairness and justice in the treatment of workers
- achieving responsibility and accountability in the workplace
- minimizing the risk of necessary but hazardous work

Occupational health issues became so fundamental to working life that they have become significant social and political issues in countries with progressive policies and a tradition of social responsibility. Issues of occupational health are deeply rooted in society and have a profound but largely unacknowledged effect on socio-economic development. According to Guidotti (2011), some of these issues include the following:

- The health risks that workers take to earn a living.
- The consequences to their families when workers become ill or injured.
- The cost of providing benefits and wage replacement to workers who are injured.
- The cost of providing medical and rehabilitation care to injured workers.
- The hidden cost to the health care system of illnesses that are not recognized as occupational, especially those that take a long time to develop.
- The loss of productivity that results from avoidable injuries and illness.
- The development of new technology, the cost of production, and return on investment.
- The social contract between workers and employers and the responsibility to keep the workplace safe.
- The financial loss to workers and their families from a prolonged illness or disabling injury.
- The social management of risk spreading, for example, by workers' compensation or other insurance plans.
- Management of and minimization of the risk of disasters.

There are five basic principles which have been identified as the basis for successful occupational health systems, as determined in a WHO/EURO survey of legislation in European countries concerning occupational health services (Rantanen, 1990). The balance among the five principles in different economic sectors, different countries, and different enterprises may vary substantially depending on the national and local conditions, traditions, laws, and practice. According to Guidotti, these five principles are as follows:

(i) Protection and Prevention

The core of occupational health activities is the principle of protection and prevention and includes the following:

- Identification of hazardous exposures and factors causing overload or other adverse work conditions;
- Assessment of the distribution and levels of exposures, identification of exposed groups or individuals, and sources of hazards;

- Assessment of risks to health and safety from exposures or adverse conditions;
- Initiating, instituting, and advising on needs and means for preventive and control actions aimed at protecting worker's health and safety.

(ii) Adaptation

All workers have not equal work ability, health status, or competence. Thus, adolescents and young workers, pregnant women, handicapped workers, ageing workers, migrant workers, and workers with chronic diseases may need adaptation of work, working methods, or work environment, including machinery and tools, to their special needs and abilities. Occupational health experts need to balance job demands with the special health and safety concerns of such workers, initiate and advise about work adaptations, and monitor the impact of such measures.

(iii) Promotion and Development

Optimally organized work can have a positive effect on workers' health and work ability: it can develop physical, mental, and professional capacities, and it can contribute to the development of safe working practices and healthy lifestyles. This principle has become especially important for industrialized countries given their attention to maintaining work ability in ageing workers, ensuring their continued participation in the workforce.

(iv) Cure and Rehabilitation

Despite the efforts for prevention and protection of work-related diseases, accidents, states of physical and mental overload and acute and chronic illnesses do occur among a substantial proportion of the workforce. An ageing working population suffers an increased risk of chronic disease conditions. The curative and rehabilitation principle is important to minimize the consequences of such events to facilitate a return to original health and work ability and, if that is not possible, to maintain the remaining work ability as much as possible.

(v) Primary Health Care

Some countries and employers include a role for primary care or general practitioner-level health care as part of occupational health services. In many countries, workers may not have access to anything but primary health care. In all countries, certain economic sectors, such as agriculture, small-scale enterprises, informal workers, home workers, and workers in remote and sparsely populated areas, usually lack specialized occupational health services and depend on primary care providers. Some countries avoid overlap and have even prohibited the combination of general health services with occupational health services. They do this to emphasize a preventive approach and to keep the management of occupational injuries and illnesses without bias. However, there are many good reasons for integrating occupational health services into primary care, which are as follows:

- To provide primary health care services, for example, injury care, quickly and conveniently at the workplace or nearby.
- To fill possible holes in public primary health services.
- To use public services most efficiently.
- To obtain a comprehensive picture of the total health of workers in the community (i.e., occupational health and general health) by capturing information at the primary care level.

Park (2009) has mentioned the factors and hazards that operate at the place of work. These factors include the following:

Physical factors: (a) Noise: Noise is a health hazard in many industries. The effects of noise are temporary or permanent hearing loss, nervousness, fatigue, decreased efficiency, etc. (b) Ultraviolet radiations: Occupations in such places effects on eyes, causing intense conjunctivitis. (c) Heat and cold: The common physical hazard in most industries is heat. The direct effects of heat exposure are burns, heat exhaustion, heat stroke, and heat cramps; the indirect effects are decreased efficiency, increased fatigue, and enhanced accident rates. Important hazards associated with cold work are chilblains, immersion foot, etc. (d) Light: The workers may be exposed to the risk of poor illumination or excessive brightness. The effects of poor illumination and excessive brightness are eye strain, headache, eye pain, eye fatigue, and discomfort visual fatigue. (e) Heat radiations. (f) Vibrations and ionizing radiations, etc.

Chemical factors: (a) Number of chemicals which cause dermatitis, eczema, ulcers, and even cancers. (b) Toxic dusts mainly cause pneumoconiosis. The most common dust diseases in our country are silicosis and anthracosis. (c) Exposure to gases such as carbon monoxide, cyanide gas, sulphur dioxide, and chlorine has a profound effect on the health of the workers. Some chemical agents cause respiratory illness, some cause injury to skin and some may have harmful effect on the blood and other organs of the body.

Biological factors: Viral, bacterial, and parasitic agents, which may result from close contact with animals or their products, contaminated water, soil, or food. The occupational diseases in this category are TB, anthrax, hydatidosis, tetanus, fungal infections, and a host of others.

Psychosocial factors that operate at the place of work are the human relationships among workers themselves on the one hand and those in authority over them on the other. Examples of psychosocial factors include the type and rhythm of work, work stability and service conditions, job satisfaction, leadership style, insecurity, workers participation, communication, system of payment, welfare conditions, degree of responsibility, trade union activities, incentives and the host of similar other factors, all entering the field of human relationships, etc. The health effects can be classified in two main categories: (a) psychological and behavioural changes: including hostility, aggressiveness, anxiety, depression, alcoholism, drug abuse, sickness, and (b) psychosomatic ill health: including fatigue, headache, hypertension, heart diseases, and rapid ageing.

Occupational hazards of agriculture workers: The health problems of workers in agriculture sector are: (a) respiratory diseases such as bagassosis, byssinosis, farmer's lung, and occupational asthma are caused by the exposure of workers to dusts of grains, rice, husks, tea, tobacco, cotton, hay, etc., (b) zoonotic diseases, such as brucellosis, anthrax, tetanus, TBs, are caused by the close contact of the agriculture workers with animals or their products, (c) toxic hazards of workers are caused by using fertilizers, insecticides, or pesticides, (d) agriculture accidents are becoming more frequent, even in developing countries, as a result of increasing use of agriculture machinery. Insect and snake bites are additional problem in India. (e) physical hazards of agriculture workers include climate conditions such as temperature, humidity, solar radiations, which may impose additional stresses upon them.

All these hazards have a profound effect upon workers everyday life. This can be seen that when a worker becomes injured or involved in any kind of disease, he becomes unable to play his normal social roles, that is, he becomes dysfunctional for his family as well as for his society. His injury or disease does not affect him alone but also his family members, who are directly or indirectly dependent on him, as well as others related to him.

Workers in the agricultural and unorganized sectors have not been covered under specific health care programmes. The increasing use of mechanization; induction of poorly trained workers who operate machines with which they are not familiar with; and the use of insecticides, pesticides, and chemicals by persons who are ignorant of the precautions to be taken are resulting in increasing health hazards to workers in these sectors. The ninth plan had recommended continuous monitoring of the safety of the work environment and workers' health status in industry and agriculture and special attention to the health problems of vulnerable groups such as women and children with a focus on the prevention, early detection, and prompt treatment. Not much progress was achieved during the ninth plan. During the tenth plan, the focus was on establishment of norms for work environment in organized, unorganized, and agricultural sectors; monitoring the work environment for detection and correction of micro environmental pollution; monitoring of health status of workers; and interventions aimed at prevention, early detection, and effective management of health problems of workers, including occupational health problems, with special attention to health problems in women and children (NCMEH, 2005).

Measures for the Health Promotion of Workers

The ILO/WHO committee on occupational health in 1953 recommended several measures for the health promotion of workers. Some specific measures, applicable in India, are given here:

- *Nutrition:* Under the Indian Factories Act, it is obligatory to provide a canteen when the number of employees exceeds 250. The aim is to provide balanced diets or snacks at reasonable cost under sanitary control.
- *Communicable disease control:* The industry should provide an excellent opportunity for early diagnosis, treatment, prevention, and rehabilitation. The communicable diseases of special importance in India are TB, typhoid, fever, malaria, and vernal diseases, etc. There should be an adequate immunization programme against preventable communicable diseases.
- *Environmental sanitation:* Within the industrial establishment, there is the need for the prevention of the spread of communicable diseases by water, food, toilet, improper ventilation, temperature, lightening, etc.
- *Measures for women and children:* Following types of measures are available for women workers in India: (a) expectant mothers are given maternity leave for 12 weeks and getting payment as per Maternity Benefit Act, (b) provision of free antenatal, natal, and postnatal services, (c) the Factories Act (section 66) prohibits night work between 7 pm and 6 am, (d) the Indian Mines Act (1923) prohibits work underground, and (e) the Factories Acts 1948 and 1976 prohibit the employment of women and children under certain occupations and below the specified age mentioned by the Constitution.
- *Health education:* Health education is a basic health need. It is an important health promotional measure. Health education in the industrial and factory setting should be envisaged at all levels—the management, the supervisory staff, the worker, and the trade union leaders of the community.
- *Family planning:* It is now recognized as a decisive factor for the quality of life and this applies to industrial workers also. The workers must adopt the small family norm.
- *Basic health goods (BHGs):* As argued by the author at different places, BHGs are the foundation of sound health. Even within the occupational environment, BHGs are important component of health.

A number of inquiries have been conducted and reports have been submitted to the government of India by many experts to protect the health condition of the workers. Park (2009) has included some of the reports in this regard: Adarkar's Report on Health Insurance for Industrial Workers (1945); Report of the Health Survey and Development Committee (1946); Report of the Health of Industrial Workers (1946); and Report of the Health of Workers in Plantation. At present, there is no comprehensive occupational health service in India. However, there are various organizations, such as organization of the chief adviser of factories, factory inspection and advisory service (1945), etc., which are active in the field of occupational health.

References

Guidotti, T. (ed.). (2011). *Global Occupational Health*, New York/New Delhi: Oxford University Press.

McKenzie, J.F., Pinger, R.R. And Kotecki, J.E. (2005). *An Introduction to Community Health*, London: Jones and Bartlett Publishers.

NCMEH. (2005). *Report of the National Commission on Macroeconomics and Health, Ministry of Health and Family Welfare*, August, Government of India, New Delhi.

Park, K. (2009). *Preventive and Social Medicine* 20th edition, Jabalpur: Banarsidas Bhanot.

Rantanen, J. ed. (1990). *Occupational Health Services: An Overview*, Copenhagen: WHO European Region

Tillman, C. (ed.). (2007). *Principles of Occupational Health and Hygiene: An Introduction*, Australia: Allen & Unwin Publication.

White, K. (2006). *SAGE Dictionary of Health and Society*, New Delhi: Sage Publications.

Chapter Twelve

Nutrition, Food and Water

'The right to food is a human right. The right to food is to ensure that all people have the capacity to feed themselves in dignity' (Gandhi, et al., 2011: 121). In other words, 'the right to adequate food is realized when every man, woman, and child, alone and in community with others, has physical and economic access at all times to adequate food or means for its procurement' (UNHCHR in Gandhi, et al., 2011: 121). It is important to note here that although food and nutrition are indispensable for every human being, sociological studies are very few in this regard. Hence, this chapter makes use of the findings of 'India Human Development Report: Towards Social Inclusion' (Gandhi, et al., 2011) for basic understanding on the issue. It is also using information provided by some of the websites and online literature for making them accessible to the readers. Food has been a basic part of our existence. Through the centuries we have acquired a wealth of information about the use of food to ensure growth of children and youth, to maintain good health through life, to meet special needs of pregnancy and lactation, and to use it to recover from illness. Food, nutrition, and health are intimately connected aspects of our life.

Let us start our study by defining these and related terms. Food nourishes the body. Food may also be defined as anything eaten or drunk, which meets the needs for energy, building, regulation, and protection of the body. In short, food is the raw material from which our bodies are made. Intake of the right kinds and amounts of food can ensure good nutrition and health, which may be evident in our appearance, efficiency, and emotional well-being (see, www.newagepublishers.com/samplechapter/000315.pdf).

Nutrition has been defined as food at work in the body. Nutrition includes everything that happens to food from the time it is eaten until it is used for various functions in the body. Nutrients are components of food that are needed by the body in adequate amounts in order to grow, reproduce, and lead a normal, healthy life. Nutrients include water, proteins, fats, carbohydrates, minerals, and vitamins. There are several nutrients in each of the groups: proteins, fats, carbohydrates, minerals, and vitamins; hence, the plural form of these words has been used. Thus, there are over 40 essential nutrients supplied by food, which are used to produce literally thousands of substances necessary for life and physical fitness. Adequate, optimum, and good nutrition are expressions used to indicate that the supply of the essential nutrients is correct in amount and proportion. It also implies that the utilization of such nutrients in the body is such that the highest level of physical and mental health is maintained throughout the life cycle.

Food has always been a central part of our social existence. It has been a part of our community, social, cultural, and religious life. Special foods are distributed as a benediction or *prasad* in the religious functions in homes, temples, and churches. Feasts are given at specific stages of life such as birth, naming ceremony, birthdays, marriages, etc. Most of the religious festivals also call for feasts and feeding of specific segments of the population. Certain menus are associated with most of these feasts in each region. Food has been used as an expression of love, friendship, and social acceptance. It is also used as a symbol of happiness at certain events in life, for example, *pedhas* are distributed to announce success in examinations, or the birth of a baby; *laddus* are associated with the celebration of Deepavali and marriages, cakes are associated with Christmas and birthdays and *tilgul* with *Sankranti*, the festival of friendship. As food is an integral part of our social existence, this function is important in daily life.

Nutrition has major effects on health. Nutrition refers to the availability of energy and nutrients to the body's cells in relation to body requirements. Malnutrition refers to any imbalance in satisfying nutrition requirements. Malnutrition among children is often caused by the synergistic effects of inadequate or improper food intake, repeated episodes of parasitic or other childhood diseases such as diarrhoea, and improper care during illness. Malnutrition is often cited as an important factor contributing to high morbidity and mortality among children in developing countries. Malnutrition during childhood can also affect growth potential and risk of morbidity and mortality in later years of life. Malnourished children are more likely to grow into malnourished adults who face increased risks of disease and death. Poor nutritional status of women has been associated with a higher age at menarche (see, for details, Mishra, Lahiri, and Luther, 1999).

A number of factors affect child nutrition, either directly or indirectly. The most commonly cited factors are food availability and dietary intake, breastfeeding, prevalence of infectious and parasitic diseases, access to health care, immunization against major childhood diseases, vitamin A supplementation, maternal care during pregnancy, water supply and sanitation, socio-economic status, and health-seeking behaviour. Demographic characteristics such as the child's age and sex, birth intervals (both preceding and following), and mother's age at childbirth are also associated with child nutrition.

Nirupam Bajpai and Ravindra H. Dholakia (2011) pointed out that India has more hungry people than any other country in the world has. The IFPRI 2010 Global Hunger Index (GHI) designates national levels of hunger as alarming, and India scores lower than many sub-Saharan African countries despite having a higher GDP. Millennium Development Goal 1 aims to halve the proportion of people suffering from hunger and indicators include (a) percentage of children under five who are underweight, and (b) proportion of the population below minimum level of dietary energy consumption. India is widely expected to miss the MDG hunger target by a significant margin.

Indicators of child and maternal undernutrition are particularly dismal. As per the WHO's standards, 40 per cent of Indian children under the age of 3 are underweight, 45 per cent are stunted, and 23 per cent have wasting. The percentage of women who are underweight decreased only marginally, from 36.2 per cent to 33 per cent, during the same period. More than 75 per cent of the population lives in households with per capita calorie consumption less than the daily minimum requirements. Nutrition interventions are spread among several government programmes and social safety nets, including the Integrated Child Development Services (ICDS) programme, the Public Distribution System (PDS), the Midday Meal Scheme (MMS), the Total Sanitation Campaign (TCS), and some activities within National Rural Health Mission (NRHM). However, India lacks a comprehensive, national nutrition strategy—and linkages between planning, managing, and implementing these interventions are often weak or ineffective.

An international comparison of India's hunger indicators presents a dismal picture. As quoted in the Nutrition Report of 2009 of the National Family and Health Survey–3 (NFHS–3), the average percentage of undernourished children under five years for 26 sub-Saharan African countries was 25 per cent, about half the Indian average of 46 per cent. Except for Kerala, Himachal Pradesh, Punjab, Sikkim, Manipur, and Mizoram, all the Indian states were either at par or worse than sub-Saharan African countries' average. Weight and height of Indians on average have not shown significant improvement over the last 25 years. A staggering 21.5 per cent of babies in India are born with low-birth weight, a problem that begins in the womb. The average per capita calorie intake was already below the minimum nutritional level of 2,400 in rural areas and 2,100 in urban areas a quarter of a century ago (1983–84). Since then, there has been a decline in per capita consumption of calories, as shown by NSS data in 1993–84 as well as 2004–05. Moreover, there has also been a consistent decline in the per capita consumption of proteins since 1983–84. It is hardly surprising then that nutritional outcome indicators for both children and adults are low and have hardly improved over the past two decades. In some states, the status of hunger and malnutrition is very worrisome. In 12 of 17 major states, the condition is 'alarming' as stated in an International Food Policy Research Institute (IFPRI) report of 2009. A third of India's adult population has a body mass index (BMI) of less than 18.5 (the number below which people are declared malnourished). The percentage of women having a BMI < 18.5 in poorer states (except Orissa) recorded a slight improvement between 1998–99 and 2005–06. Socially marginalized castes/tribes also have a higher percentage of women with BMI < 18.5 (India Human Development Report: Towards Social Inclusion).

Malnutrition in India

Malnutrition is a serious problem, especially for infants and young children. It reflects an imbalance of both macro- and micro-nutrients that may be due to inappropriate intake and/or inefficient biological utilization due to the internal and external environment. Poor feeding practices during infancy and early childhood, resulting in malnutrition, contribute to impaired cognitive and social development, poor school performance, and reduced productivity in later life. Malnutrition, therefore, is a major threat to social and economic development as it is among the most serious obstacles to attaining and maintaining the health of this important age group. According to the United Nations Standing Committee on Nutrition, 2006, undernutrition is the main threat to health and well-being not only in middle- and low-income countries but also globally (Global Hunger Index, GHI, 2010).

Lack of essential nutrients and insufficient calories can be extremely detrimental to their early growth and development and cannot always be reversed with improved dietary intake. While commonly associated with poverty and a deprived environment, not all malnutrition results from a shortage of money. Children of middle- and upper-income families may also be malnourished because of unwise food selections. Frequent fast food meals, snacking habits, concern over weight control, and skipped meals can seriously limit the variety of food choices, which, in turn, limit the nutrients ingested (Moran, 1999). Some children also experience malnutrition as a result of certain health conditions and disease (visit for details http://webtools.delmarlearning.com/sample_chapters/marotz_ch01.pdf).

Over half (54%) of all childhood deaths in India are related to malnutrition. Nearly 30 per cent of the global childhood deaths attributed to stunting, severe wasting, and intrauterine growth restriction—low-birth weight occur in India. In 2005–06, about 44 per cent of Indian children under 5 were underweight, and 48 per cent were stunted due to chronic malnutrition. Due to the country's size, this means India is home to 42 per cent of the world's underweight children and 31 per cent of the world's stunted children. The proportion of stunted and undernourished children is 19–21 times higher than expected for a healthy, well-nourished population according to international child growth standards.

High levels of child undernutrition are driven by the low nutritional and social status of women. Forty per cent of women in India have low body mass, a factor in low-birth weight. Twenty-eight per cent of children born in India are low-birth weight, indicating intrauterine undernutrition. Nearly half of low-birth-weight babies are currently stunted or underweight, compared to one-third of normal birth weight babies. Nearly 40 per cent of all low-birth-weight babies in the world are born in India. Undernutrition indicators in India also follow lines of inequity—undernutrition is substantially higher in rural areas than in urban areas, and children from scheduled tribes have the poorest nutritional status on nearly every measure and the highest prevalence of wasting (28%) among under-fives.

The proportion of severely underweight children is nearly five times higher among children whose mothers have no education than mothers who have 12 or more years of school. However, undernutrition is a considerable issue even among wealthier families; even in households within the highest wealth quintile, 25 per cent of children are stunted and 20 per cent are underweight. This points to widespread poor feeding practices in India, particularly during the 1,000–day window of opportunity from conception until the child's second birthday. NFHS–3 reports that while breastfeeding is nearly universal, it is not done correctly. Only 25 per cent of newborns breastfed within 1 hour of birth, less than half of infants under six months were exclusively breastfed, and only 20 per cent of children 6–23 months of age are fed according to recommended practices.

Female malnutrition among the SCs and STs is higher than the national average; it is even worse in the low per capita income states (Bihar and Orissa) even within these groups. Further, female malnutrition among SCs and STs has been increasing over the years. The highest percentage of underweight and stunted children was recorded for STs (54.5% and 53.9%, respectively) followed by SCs (47.9% and 53.9%, respectively). Children belonging to the STs had the highest percentage suffering from anaemia in 2005–06, followed by SCs. Among both SCs and STs, a high percentage of children suffering from anaemia hail from states with a low per capita income, namely, West Bengal, Madhya Pradesh, Uttar Pradesh, Orissa, Jharkhand, Chhattisgarh, and Bihar.

We have discussed the issue even elsewhere, but it is relevant to quote here that the observation made by the High Level Expert Group (HLEG) constituted by Government of India, in 2011, for suggesting a new model of Universal Health Coverage (UHC). It says, more than a fourth of the world's population who are hungry are Indians. As per the WHO's standards, 40 per cent of Indian children under the age of 3 are underweight, 45 per cent are stunted, and 23 per cent have wasting. Malnutrition itself is the result of several other determinants that have extended and extenuating lifetime impact on the health and well-being of women and their children. Even economically developed states—Gujarat, Maharashtra, Andhra Pradesh, and Karnataka—have high levels of food insecurity. However, there are states that have taken initiative to combat the challenge. Government of Bihar's recent decision to set up a Human Development Mission under the Chief Minister, with 12–14 well-defined outcomes, and each having 2–5 process indicators with agreed means of verification, is a very good step in the right direction. There is a need to adopt a human development approach to fight malnutrition and anaemia. It is time to shed narrow departmentalism and petty turf issues; malnutrition is not a department's mandate—it is a government's mandate!! 'Nayi Pidhi Swasthya Guarantee Karyakram', which was launched by the Government of Bihar to cover each and every 3.4 crore boys (0–14 age) and girls (0–18 age) for health check up, health card, and complete referral follow-up, is also an effective way of reaching to every child and girl adolescent in order to decrease the rate of malnutrition, anaemia, and low-age marriage.

Nutritional status affects children's behaviour too. Well-nourished children are more alert, attentive, and better able to benefit from physical activity and learning experiences. Poorly nourished children may be quiet and withdrawn, or hyperactive and disruptive during class activities. Children who are overweight also face many social, emotional, and physical problems. They are often slow and less able to participate in physical activity. They may also suffer ridicule, emotional stress, and be excluded from their peer groups. Children's resistance to infection and illness is also directly influenced by their nutritional status. Children who are well nourished are less likely to become ill; they also recover more quickly when they are sick. Poorly nourished children are more susceptible to infections and illness, while illness increases the need for some nutrients. Thus, poor nutrition creates a cycle of illness, poorer nutritional status, and lowered resistance to illness.

Water

According to Kofi Annan, for UN General Secretary, 'Access to safe water is a fundamental human need and, therefore, a basic human right. Contaminated water jeopardizes both the physical and social health of all people. It is an affront to human dignity'. Water is the essence of life. Without water, human beings cannot live for more than a few days. It plays a vital role in nearly every function of the body, protecting the immune system—the body's natural defences—and helping remove waste matter. But to do this effectively, water must be accessible and safe. 'Lack of safe water is a cause of serious illnesses such as diarrhoeal diseases, which kill over 2 million people every year (the vast majority children, mostly in developing countries). Contaminated water, whether drunk or used to cook food, harms people's health. Water is also essential for hygiene, growing food, keeping animals, rest, exercise, and relaxation and for a variety of social and cultural reasons (WHO, 2003: 6).

Although water is indispensable for human or animal or even biological life cycle, studies on availability, accessibility, and affordability of safe or potable drinking water are rare. WHO has studied the water issue at length and this chapter is using most of the WHO literature for having a proper and authentic understanding on the issue. Access to a regular supply of safe water is a basic human right, as is access to unadulterated food. But as with other human rights, too many people miss out. Of the world's population of 6 billion people, at least 1.1 billion do not have available sources of clean drinking water, such as protected springs and wells. Lack of access to safe water has a major effect on people's health. Poor health constrains development and poverty alleviation. Poor water and sanitation have an impact on education, but when safe water and appropriate sanitation are provided in schools, there is an increase in attendance and a reduction in drop-out rates.

General comment 15, on the right to water, adopted in November 2002 by the Committee on Economic, Social and Cultural Rights (ESCR), sets the criteria for the full enjoyment of the right to water. More than 1 billion people lack access to improved sources of drinking water, and all of them suffer the consequences—health problems, economic and social difficulties, and inequities. Certain groups are affected in a specific and dramatic way. Further, the observation made by the High Level Expert Group (HLEG) constituted in 2011 for suggesting a new model of Universal Health Coverage (UHC) says that there is a clear correlation between inadequate and poor quality of water or sanitation and health. A study of urban poor communities in Mumbai found that water-related illnesses accounted for almost a third of all morbidity in the last year among adults, and almost two-thirds of all morbidity among children. Another study in five Indian states found a negative correlation between the provision of household toilets and community-level prevalence of communicable diseases including cholera, typhoid/enteric disease, diarrhoea/vomiting, hepatitis, nematodal infections as well as malaria and dengue. A 2002 Planning Commission report expressed alarm over the 'rather extensive presence' of fluoride and arsenic in Indian drinking water, which is associated with a number of cancers (of the skin, lungs, kidneys, and bladder). According to the Water and Sanitation Programme, the cost per Disability Adjusted Life Year (DALY) of poor sanitation in urban areas is estimated at 5,400 INR.

The Poor

Among those most directly affected by unsafe water are the poor in both rural and urban areas. Not only are the poor less likely to have access to safe water and sanitation, but they are also less likely to have the financial and human resources to manage the impact of this deprivation. Some 80 per cent of those who have no access to improved sources of drinking water are the rural poor—who may also have less access to political and lobbying processes than their urban counterparts. The 'cost' of lack of access to safe water is reflected in the day-to-day investment of time to collect water—time that is not then available for productive activity, household, or child care or education—and in the burden of disease arising from water collection—including injury and water contact diseases such as schistosomiasis. In many cities, the poorest residents live in shanty towns and slums, sometimes on the edge of the city. These settlements generally lie outside formal water and sanitation distribution networks. They are often not recognized by the city authorities, who may not support extension of essential services, whether public or private, to these areas. Poor families without access to safe water frequently find themselves even poorer as a result of ill health caused by the lack of safe water.

Children

The Convention on the Rights of the Child, 1989, in Article 24, obliges states parties to pursue full implementation of the right to the highest standard of attainable health and, in particular, to take appropriate measures to provide adequate nutritious foods and clean drinking water, taking into consideration the dangers and risks of environmental pollution. The lack of accessible safe water increases the vulnerability of children to diseases. Their immune systems and detoxification mechanisms are not fully developed, so they are often less able to respond to a water-related infection.

Indigenous Peoples

Indigenous peoples may face problems accessing safe water. Natural water sources traditionally used by them, such as lakes and rivers, may no longer be accessible because of land expropriation or contamination. While water is important to every community, many indigenous groups rely on waterways and water bodies for their traditional livelihoods, including fishing, whaling, and sealing. When access to fresh water is compromised, often indigenous rights to self-determination and occupation are impinged upon, as are their water-reliant traditions.

Thus, the governments hold the primary responsibility for ensuring the realization of human rights. The United Nations Committee on Economic, Social and Cultural Rights has stated that governments have a number of duties to follow from the right to water. Governments must take the steps necessary to ensure that everyone can enjoy sufficient, safe, acceptable, accessible, and affordable water, without discrimination. While some discretion is allowed in the choice and mix of the measures to be taken—for example, law, policies, and programmes—they must be targeted and directed towards full implementation of the right.

We can conclude this discussion with the remarks of the High Level Expert Group Report on Universal Health Coverage for India (HLEG, 2011) constituted by Government of India: There is a clear correlation between inadequate and poor quality of water or sanitation and health. A study of urban poor communities in Mumbai found that water-related illnesses accounted for almost a third of all morbidity in the last year among adults, and almost two-thirds of all morbidity among children. Another study in five Indian states found a negative correlation between the provision of household toilets and community-level prevalence of communicable diseases including cholera, typhoid/enteric disease, diarrhoea/vomiting, hepatitis, nematodal infections as well as malaria and dengue. A 2002 Planning Commission report expressed alarm over the 'rather extensive presence' of fluoride and arsenic in Indian drinking water, which is associated with a number of cancers (of the skin, lungs, kidneys, and bladder). According to the Water and Sanitation Programme, the cost per Disability Adjusted Life Year (DALY) of poor sanitation in urban areas is estimated at 5,400 INR. Another major finding is that use of improved facilities is strongly correlated with sanitation related knowledge and hygiene-promotive attitudes.

References

Bajpai, N. and Dholakia, R.H. (2011). *Improving the Integration of Health and Nutrition Sectors in India*, Columbia Global Centres/South Asia, Columbia University.

Gandhi, A., Kumar, C., Saha, P., Sahoo, B.K. and Sharma, A. (2011). *India Human Development Report; Towards Social Inclusion*, Institute of Applied Manpower Research, Planning commission, Government of India, Oxford University Press, New Delhi.

Global Hunger Index: The Challenge of Hunger: Focus on the Crisis of Child Undernutrition. (2010). International Food Policy Research Institute, Concern Worldwide and Welthungerhilfe. Available online at: www.ifpri.org/publication/2010–global-hunger-index.

HLEG. (2011). *Report of the High Level Expert Group on Universal Health Coverage,* Planning Commission, Government of India. Available online at: http://planningcommission.nic.in/reports/genrep/rep_uhc0812.pdf.

Mishra, V.K., Lahiri, S. and Luther, N.Y. (1999). Child Nutrition in India, National Family Health Survey Subject Reports, Number 14, June International Institute for Population Sciences Mumbai, India, pp. 5–6.

Moran, R. (1999). 'Evaluation and treatment of childhood obesity', *American Family Physician,* 59, 861. Cited in http://webtools.delmarlearning.com/sample_chapters/marotz_ch01.pdf

World Health Organization. (2003). *Right to Water,* Health and Human Rights Publication Series; no. 3, World Health Organization. http://webtools.delmarlearning.com/sample_chapters/marotz_ch01.pdf

CHAPTER THIRTEEN

Sanitation and Environment

The word 'sanitation' is derived from the Latin word *Sanitas,* which means a state of health. It comprises all interventions which aim to protect and promote human health by providing a clean environment and breaking the cycle of disease. It refers to the principles and practices relating to the collection, treatment, removal or disposal of human excreta, household wastewater, and refuse as they impact upon people and the environment (Müllegger, Langergraber and Lechner, 2011). The World Health Organization states that:

> Sanitation generally refers to the provision of facilities and services for the safe disposal of human urine and feces. Inadequate sanitation is a major cause of disease world-wide and improving sanitation is known to have a significant beneficial impact on health both in households and across communities. The word 'sanitation' also refers to the maintenance of hygienic conditions, through services such as garbage collection and wastewater disposal. (http://www.who.int/topics/sanitation/en/)

The term 'sanitation' can be applied to a specific aspect, concept, location, or strategy, such as:

- Improved sanitation—refers to the management of human faeces at the household level. This terminology is the indicator used to describe the target of the millennium development goal on sanitation, by the WHO/UNICEF joint monitoring programme for water supply and sanitation.
- On-site sanitation—the collection and treatment of waste is done where it is deposited. Examples are the use of pit latrines, septic tanks, and Imhoff tanks.
- Food sanitation—refers to the hygienic measures for ensuring food safety.
- Environmental sanitation—the control of environmental factors that form links in disease transmission. Subsets of this category are solid waste management, water and wastewater treatment, industrial waste treatment and noise and pollution control.
- Ecological sanitation—an approach that tries to emulate nature through the recycling of nutrients and water from human and animal wastes in a hygienically safe manner (see, for details, en.wikipedia.org/wiki/Sanitation).

Elke Müllegger, Günter Langergraber and Markus Lechner of EcoSan Club have discussed the issue of sanitation at length. This chapter has used their views for understanding various issues. There are 2.6 billion people who are living without adequate sanitation; the vast majority of population are in India, China, and Africa. Progress in provision of sanitation services is struggling to keep up with population growth, and Africa is lagging behind the most. Within 20 years, it is expected that an additional 2 billion will live in towns and cities demanding sanitation. The challenge is obvious, already today sanitation-related diseases and poor hygienic conditions cause 2.2 million deaths annually (mostly children under the age of 5). Other consequences are the massive pollution of water and soil, the loss of innumerable school—(mainly girls) and working days, losses in tourism income, prevention of economic growth, etc.

In order to be sustainable, a sanitation system has to be not only economically viable, socially acceptable, and technically and institutionally appropriate, but it should also protect the environment and the natural resources. Thus, sustainability in the sanitation sector refers to five interrelated dimensions: technical, financial, institutional, social, and environmental. The Sustainable Sanitation Alliance (SSA) links these sustainability criteria to the following aspects:

- *Health and hygiene:* includes the risk of exposure to human pathogens and hazardous substances; hygiene, nutrition and improvement of livelihood; effects on the health of downstream populations.
- *Environment and natural resources:* involves the required energy, water, and other natural resources; the potential emissions to the environment resulting from their use, the degree of recycling practiced, and their effects.
- *Technology and operation:* incorporates the functionality and the ease of construction, operation, maintenance, and monitoring; suitability to achieve an efficient substance flow management; robustness as well as flexibility and adaptability of the system.
- *Financial and economic issues:* relates to the capacity of households and communities to pay for sanitation; economic benefits from the production of the recyclables, employment creation, increased productivity through improved health, and the reduction of environmental and public health costs.
- *Socio-cultural and institutional aspects:* includes the socio-cultural acceptance and appropriateness of the system; convenience; gender issues and impacts on human dignity; the contribution to subsistence economies and food security; and legal and institutional aspects.

The sanitation crisis is keenly felt in informal settlements across the globe. With no way to safely dispose either faeces or garbage, around a billion slum dwellers must resort to 'flying toilets' (plastic bags that are used then thrown away) and to dumping trash in public spaces. This situation is not limited to urban settlements; in impoverished city suburbs, small market towns, large villages, and periurban settlements across the developing world, the public environment is full of human wastes. The contents of bucket-latrines and pits, even of sewers, are often emptied into the streets, lakes, rivers, or coasts. This excrement immediately contaminates the surrounding environment, enters waterways, and harms communities (see, Sanitation-sustains-clean-environments. Available at www.unicef.org.mz/claudio/f5_environment.pdf).

Water and sanitation are environmental issues to their very core, and together constitute one of the top drivers of development. Managing water supplies so that they become neither depleted nor polluted and providing good sanitation are central to the health of communities and the environment on which they depend. Poor water and sanitation provision can affect entire communities: one person's bad sanitation is another's contaminated food or water. Even piped systems, if poorly managed, can concentrate any 'downstream' problems—such as pollution in rivers, lakes, and seas—and further degrade wildlife habitats and contribute to human health problems. Where water and sanitation deficiencies are severe, there are likely to be a range of serious public health hazards (Environment, Water and Sanitation, Irish Aid key sheet, Environment Policy for Sustainable Development, www.irishaid.gov.ie).

The term 'environmental sanitation' has been given various interpretations in different countries and at different times. In its most restrictive sense, sanitation has been equated with the safe disposal of human excrement. Environmental sanitation is a major public health issue in India. Recent interventional studies on environmental sanitation in India highlighted the importance of prioritizing control strategies. Research related to the appropriate cost-effective intervention strategies and their implementation in Indian context is a big challenge.

Environmental sanitation means the control of all those factors in man's surroundings, which may or may not cause adverse effects on his health. The sanitarian makes an effort towards hygiene of water supply and food supply, hygienic disposal of human and animal wastes, hygiene of housing, and control of rodents and other vectors (RSHB). The World Health Organization (WHO) defines 'environmental sanitation' as 'the control of all those factors in man's physical environment which exercise or may exercise a deleterious effect on his physical development, health and survival'. Environmental sanitation/hygiene includes all the activities aimed at improving or maintaining the standard of basic environmental conditions affecting the well-being of people. These conditions include the following:

- Clean and safe water supply
- Clean and safe ambient air

- Efficient and safe animal, human, and industrial waste disposal
- Protection of food from biological and chemical contaminants
- Adequate housing in clean and safe surroundings (http://www.healthizen.com/blog/index.php/general/environmental-sanitation/)

According to P.C. Mmom and C.F. Mmom (2011), environmental sanitation comprises disposal and treatment of human excreta, solid waste and waste water, control of disease vectors, and provision of washing facilities for personal and domestic hygiene. It aims at improving the quality of life of the individuals and contributing to social development. It has been defined by the Water Supply and Sanitation Collaborative Council as 'Interventions to reduce people's exposure to disease by providing a clean environment in which to live, with measures to break the cycle of disease. Environmental sanitation comprises both a change in behaviour and facilities to form a hygienic environment. However, it is a truism that a significant number of people worldwide lack access to adequate water, sanitation, drainage, and solid waste disposal services. The latest statistics reveal that 1.1 billion people still do not have access to safe drinking water, and 2.4 billion people do not have access to adequate sanitation' (WHO/UNICEF/WSSCC, 2000, cited by Kawachi and Berkman, 2003). Furthermore, in many urban areas of developing countries, less than 50 per cent of the municipal solid wastes are collected and only an insignificant fraction is disposed of appropriately. This not only increases the rate of diseases and mortality, but also slows down the economic progress of hundreds of millions of people in developing countries. At the same time, the world's natural supply of freshwater is subject to increasing environmental and economic pressure. Mmom (2003) noted that urban environmental condition is deplorable in many cities of the developing world. In fact, the problems associated with providing environmental sanitation services are central to the urbanization phenomena. Urban waste is considered one of the most serious and pressing urban environmental problems. Most cities focus on simply getting rid of their waste 'out-of-sight' and fail to recognize its potential danger when not properly disposed, treated, or managed.

In developing countries, waste management often emerges as a problem that endangers human health and the environment. To make matters worse, waste management usually has a low priority on the political agenda of such countries, as they are struggling with other important issues such as hunger, health problems, water shortages, and unemployment. In such situations, it is easy to understand why waste problems have a tendency to grow steadily. Several past researches have focused on investigating the cost benefits of providing safe and convenient living conditions to households in the developing world, especially on housing conditions, notably on the relationship between water, sanitation, and disease. Citing from different sources, Yongsi, Herrmann, Ntetu, Sietchiping, and Herrmann (2008) state that water supply, sanitation, and health are closely related. It is also evident that each year, poor hygiene, mismanagement of liquid or solid waste, and lack of sanitation facilities contribute to the death of millions of the world's poorest people from preventable diseases. Considering the nexus of cleansing/sanitation and health, empirical evidence points to their close linkages. In particular, the relationship could be outlined as follows:

1. As cities continue to grow, the management of solid waste is becoming a major environmental and public health concern in urban areas of many developing countries.
2. Lack of sanitation and unsafe disposal or storage of waste in/around houses and streets and in undesignated containers may provide habitats for vectors of that cause various infectious diseases including amoebiasis, typhoid fever, and diarrhoeas.
3. Uncontrolled landfills are a huge danger for the surrounding environment and are a health risk to the population, causing contamination of the drinking water and soil.
4. More than 5 million people die each year from diseases related to inadequate waste disposal systems (WHO, 2007).

It is estimated that 1.8 million people die worldwide every year from diarrhoeal diseases (including cholera). Among them, 90 per cent are children under 5 mostly in developing societies. An estimated 88 per cent of this burden is attributed to unsafe drinking water supply, inadequate sanitation, and poor hygiene. These risk factors do not evenly threaten urban districts as slums and informal settlements are more vulnerable to communicable diseases (Yongsi, Herrmann, Ntetu, Sietchiping, and Herrmann, 2008).

As per estimates, inadequate sanitation costs India almost $54 billion or 6.4 per cent of the country's GDP in 2006. Over 70 per cent of this economic impact or about $38.5 billion was health related, with diarrhoea followed by acute lower respiratory infections accounting for 12 per cent of the health-related impacts. Evidence suggests that all water and sanitation improvements are cost-beneficial in the subregions of the developing world. Sectoral demands for water are growing rapidly in India owing mainly to urbanization and it is estimated that by 2025, more than 50 per cent of the country's population will live in cities and towns. Population increase, rising incomes, and industrial growth are also responsible for this dramatic shift. National Urban Sanitation Policy, 2008 was the recent development in order to rapidly promote sanitation in urban areas of the country. India's Ministry of Urban Development commissioned the survey as part of its National Urban Sanitation Policy in November 2008. In rural areas, local government institutions in charge of operating and maintaining the infrastructure are seen as weak and lack the financial resources to carry out their functions. In addition, no major city in India is known to have a continuous water supply and an estimated 72 per cent of Indians still lack access to improved sanitation facilities. Besides this, the 63 per cent of urban population in India is without proper sanitation. The 11th Five-Year Plan envisages 100 per cent coverage of urban water, urban sewerage, and rural sanitation by 2012. Although investment in water supply and sanitation is likely to see a jump of 221 per cent in the 11th plan over the 10th plan, the targets do not take into account the quality of water being provided or the sustainability of systems being put in place (Kumar, Kar, and Jain, 2011).

India is still lagging far behind many countries in the field of environmental sanitation. According to Pandve (2008), most cities and towns in India are characterized by overcrowding, congestion, inadequate water supply, and inadequate facilities of disposal of human excreta, wastewater, and solid wastes. Most of the problems in the country are due to defective environment, which in turn rob people of their health, destroy their livelihoods, and undermine their overall development potential. The environmental sanitation is still an ignored issue in India. To raise the overall of standard of living, the issue of environmental sanitation must be tackled seriously. It is essential to take some stricter steps to raise the current state of environmental sanitation in India. For example in Nigeria, the state government of Lagos has set up a sanitation court, which will prosecute offenders arrested for violating the state environmental sanitation.

The Environmental Burden of Disease

According to a study conducted by Environment and Social Development Unit South Asia Region (Environmental Health in India: Priorities in Andhra Pradesh, 2001), environmental factors account for about 20 per cent of the total burden of disease in Andhra Pradesh. Over 90 per cent of this is associated with traditional environmental risks, such as lack of access to a protected water supply and sanitation (73% of AP's population has no sanitation facilities) and indoor air pollution resulting from the use of biomass fuels. The largest portion of the environmental burden of ill health is borne by people in rural areas, where access to basic infrastructure services (water, sanitation, and commercial fuels) is lower and where baseline infant and child mortality rates are higher than in urban AP. In rural areas, environmental factors account for 22–23 per cent of the burden of disease, significantly higher than urban areas. This burden is almost entirely caused by the lack of access to water and sanitation facilities and by exposure to indoor air pollution (89% of the rural population relies on wood and dung cakes for cooking fuel) and contaminated drinking water. Thus, while modern environmental risks linked to industrial pollution and urban development also exist and are growing, environmental health is still to a large degree a rural health issue in AP—and will continue to be for quite some time. Urban households have much higher levels of access to water and sanitation services and rely less upon dirty cooking fuels. As a result of these and other factors (such as higher levels of income and education), the average burden of disease is significantly lower for the urban population, as is the share of the household environment in the total burden.

Promoting Sanitation

Many diseases are spread from person to person by germs in faeces. According to Jeff Conant (2005), some experts believe health problems from poor sanitation can be prevented only if people change their personal habits, or 'behaviours', about staying clean. But this idea often leads to failure because it does not consider the barriers that people face in their daily lives, such as poverty or lack of access to clean water. Then when behaviour does not change, people are blamed for their own poor health. Other experts look for technical solutions, such as modern toilets that flush water. Technical solutions often come from outside a community and may not fit the traditions or conditions of the community. Sometimes they create more problems than they solve! The diseases caused by germs from poor hygiene and sanitation will not be prevented if people are blamed for their own poor health, or if only technical solutions are promoted. To improve health in a lasting way, health promoters must listen carefully and work together with people in the community. When communities use hygiene and sanitation methods that fit their real needs and abilities, they will enjoy better health.

The poor sanitation leads to more health problems. Illnesses caused by germs and worms in faeces are a constant source of discomfort for millions of people. These illnesses can cause many years of sickness and can lead to other health problems such as dehydration, anaemia, and malnutrition. Severe sanitation-related illnesses such as cholera can spread rapidly, bringing sudden death to many people.

Children have a high risk of illness from poor sanitation. While adults may live with diarrhoea diseases and worms, children die from these illnesses. It is important for children to have toilets that are safe and that feel safe. When children feel safe using the toilet and have an easy way to stay clean, they get less sick. Many children, especially girls, leave school because safe toilets and healthy conditions are not provided for them. Allowing children to help build toilets and teaching them about illness caused by poor sanitation are some ways to help them develop healthy behaviours.

References

Conant, J. (2005). *Sanitation and Cleanliness for a Healthy Environment*, USA: Hesperian Foundation.

Environment, Water and Sanitation, Irish Aid key sheet, Environment Policy for Sustainable Development. Available online at: www.irishaid.gov.ie.

Environmental Health in India: Priorities in Andhra Pradesh. (2001). Environment and Social Development Unit South Asia Region, October.

Kawachi, I. and Berkman, L.F. (2003). *Neighborhoods and Health*. New York: Oxford University Press

Kumar, G.S., Kar, S.S. and Jain, A. (2011). 'Health and Environmental Sanitation in India: Issues for Prioritizing Control Strategies', *Indian Journal of Occupational and Environmental Medicine*, September 15(3): 93–96.

Mmom, P.C., (2003). 'Willingness of Port Harcourt City residents to relocate their residence; implication for urban decongestion', *J. Pedagogy Dev.*, Special Edn., pp: 78–89. Cited in Mmom, P.C. and Mmom, C.F. (2011).

Mmom, P.C. and Mmom, C.F. (2011). 'Environmental Sanitation and Public Health Challenges in A Rapidly Growing City of the Third World: The Case of Domestic Waste and Diarrhoea Incidence in Greater Port Harcourt Metropolis, Nigeria' *Asian Journal of Medical Sciences* 3(3).

Müllegger, E., Langergraber, G. and Lechner, M. (2011). 'Sustainable Sanitation Practice, Planning Tools: Sustainable Sanitation Practice', *EcoSanClub*, Issue 7. Available at: http://www.seecon.ch/sites/default/files/projects/files/spp_sswm_toolbox.pdf

Pandve, H.T. (2008). 'Environmental Sanitation: An Ignored Issue in India', *Indian Journal of Occupational and Environmental Medicine*, 12(1): 40.

Yongsi, H.B.N., Herrmann, T.M., Ntetu, A.L., Sietchiping, R. and Herrmann, C.B., (2008). 'Environmental Sanitation and Health Risks in Tropical Urban Settings: Case Study of Household Refuse and Diarrhea in YaoundéCameroon', *International Journal of Human and Social Sciences*, 3: 3, 220–228, Available at www.waset.org/journals/ijhss/v3/v3-3-29.pdf

WHO (2007). Available at:
http://www.who.int/whr/2007/ en/index.html
http://www.healthizen.com/blog/index.php/general/environmental-sanitation/whqlibdoc.who.int/publications/a38153_(ch21).pdf.
en.wikipedia.org/wiki/Sanitation.

Chapter Fourteen

Public Health, Health Structure, and Health Programmes

Health status of a population and especially of the vulnerable population is now considered an important indicator of development. Health is increasingly being seen as a development issue rather than just a medical issue. Ill health and poor access to health services are seen as indicator of poor economies and irresponsible health policies. Most governments, all over the world, are recognizing the importance of health programmes in reducing the incidences of disease, disability, premature mortality, effects of ageing, and improving the physical, mental, and socio-cultural conditions of living. Public health broadly refers to the efforts taken by the government for improving collective or community health, as a whole. The Expert Committee of WHO has defined public health as the 'science and art of preventing diseases, prolonging life, and promoting mental and physical health and efficiency through organized community efforts for the sanitation of the environment, the control of communicable infection, the education of the individual's personal hygiene, the organization of medical and nursing services for early diagnosis and preventive treatment of disease, the development of the social machinery to ensure to every individual a standard of living, adequate for the maintenance of health and so organizing these benefits as to enable every citizen to realize his birth right of health and longevity' (WHO, 1952).

J.B. Grant, in a detailed and explanatory definition states: 'Public health is the science and art of social utilization of scientific knowledge for medical protection by maintaining health, preventing disease, and curing disease through organized community efforts for (a) the hygiene of the environment, (b) the control of the community infections, (c) the education of the individual in principles of personal hygiene, (d) the organization of medical and nursing service for the early diagnosis and preventive treatment of disease, and (e) the development of social machinery which will ensure to every individual in the community a standard of living adequate for the maintenance of health. As such, public health becomes social medicine and is primarily a field of social activity, applying practically every basic science directed towards a comprehensive programme of community service' (Bagchi and Soman, 2005: 45).

The standard of health of people depends upon the levels of living, literacy, nutrition, sanitation, environment, and organization of health services which in turn depends on money, materials, and institutions. Health is a logical prerequisite for socio-economic development as it affects both productivity and production. It is an important input for the development of man and thereby to social and economic development of the country. Achievement of good health and its maintenance is one of the universal values accepted by humanity as expressed through WHO's definition of health. This has changed the focus of the western medicine from treatment-oriented, hospital-based curative medicine to community-based curative and preventive medicine. This shift has necessitated the knowledge about the community, its culture, and ways of living.

Public health systems vary in different parts of the world, depending upon the prevalent health problems. In the developing world, where sanitation problems and limited medical resources persist, infectious diseases are the most significant threat to public health. Public health officials devote resources to establish sanitation systems and immunization programmes to curb the spread of infectious diseases, and provide routine medical care to rural and isolated populations. In industrialized nations, sanitary food and water supplies and excellent medical resources have reduced rates of infectious disease. Instead, accidents and diseases such as lung cancer, heart attacks, and strokes are among the leading causes of death. In these areas, public health goals include education programmes to teach people how to prevent accidents and lessen their risk for disease, and the maintenance of the excellent disease prevention systems already established.

At the present time, the field of public health is in a state of flux, for the concerns at every level of participation have changed enormously in recent years. The traditional concerns have receded in importance, while new challenges in fields such as industrial health, nutrition, environmental pollution, accidents, insurance, health education and behaviour change, health-service research, social epidemiology and aetiology, and health care administration loom very large. The involvement of non-governmental organizations (NGOs) in health and especially public health issues are doing great jobs in creating awareness among the masses and ensuring community participation. The new studies conducted in the field of public health research and epidemiological research is giving ways to more realistic and pragmatic policy formulations. Public health plays an important role in disease prevention efforts in both the developing world and developed countries, through local health systems and non-governmental organizations.

The World Health Organization (WHO) is the international agency that coordinates and acts on global public health issues. Most countries have their own government public health agencies, sometimes known as ministries of health, to respond to domestic health issues. For example in the United States, the front line of public health initiatives is state and local health departments. The United States Public Health Service (PHS), led by the Surgeon General of the United States, and the Centers for Disease Control and Prevention, headquartered in Atlanta, are involved with several international health activities, in addition to their national duties. In Canada, the Public Health Agency of Canada is the national agency responsible for public health, emergency preparedness and response, and infectious and chronic disease control and prevention. The public health system in India is managed by the Ministry of Health and Family Welfare of the Government of India with state-owned health care facilities.

There is a vast discrepancy in access to health care and public health initiatives between developed nations and developing nations. In the developing world, public health infrastructures are still forming. There may not be enough trained health workers or monetary resources to provide even a basic level of medical care and disease prevention. As a result, a large majority of disease and mortality in the developing world results from and contributes to extreme poverty. For example, many African governments spend less than US$10 per person per year on health care, while in the United States, the federal government spent approximately US$ 4,500 per capita in 2000. However, expenditures on health care should not be confused with spending on public health. Public health measures may not generally be considered 'health care' in the strictest sense. For example, mandating the use of seat belts in cars can save countless lives and contribute to the health of a population, but typically money spent enforcing this rule would not count as money spent on health care.

In some ways, public health is a modern concept of human development in science, although it has roots in antiquity. From the beginnings of human civilization, it was recognized that polluted water and lack of proper waste disposal spread communicable diseases (theory of miasma). Early religions attempted to regulate behaviour that specifically related to health, from types of food eaten, to regulating certain indulgent behaviours, such as drinking alcohol or sexual relations. The establishment of governments placed responsibility on leaders to develop public health policies and programmes in order to gain some understanding of the causes of disease and thus ensure social stability prosperity, and maintain order.

Health systems in contemporary societies are invariably dependent upon the political economy of the systems in which they operate. Polities in modern context and especially in the democratic set-ups can no longer ignore the health prescriptions suggested by

WHO because such prescriptions also match to the felt needs and aspirations of politically conscious and numerically decisive citizens. But the delivery systems do not always reflect the political idealism of 'health for all'. Economies, in the age of globalization, look at health as the largest long-term investment for harnessing the human resources, as well as, marketing potentials. The inequalities created in political-economic systems did get reflected in terms of health opportunities and privileges.

The delivery of the health care system has to be determined by the health expectations of the people and these are also influenced by the social, cultural, economic, and situational factors in the community. In a country which has been characterized by inequalities of all sorts, seeking equilibrium between the health providers and health seekers is a great challenge. Social sciences are doing their best to create situations in which health facilities should not only be made available to the masses but also be made accessible for them. Going by the socio-cultural and economic factors of health, studies reflect that poverty continues to be the greatest hurdle in ensuring good health in developing countries. Poor health drives the poor into absolute poverty and poverty pushes them back into poor health status. Unavailability of food, malnutrition, poor sanitation, illiteracy, lack of education, inadequate and ill-constructed housing, unemployment, poor working condition, etc., are other socio-cultural factors which act as barriers in ensuring good health. Some other problems such as food adulteration, unhygienic additives, and food poisoning are some factors which target specifically the poor and the other marginalized communities (see also Akram, 2012a; Advani and Akram, 2007).

Development of Health Structure in India

Qadeer (1985) points out that the present system of health services in India is the result of attempts made by the British to make their position strong in India. The Government of India appointed various committees of experts on health in order to look properly in the health sector and suggest recommendations to overcome the health problems and improve the health status of population. The recommendations put forth by various committees are briefly discussed here as these will help us to understand the evolution of health structure in India and the inherent contradictions and biases.

Reports of Various Committees

- *The Bhore Committee (1943):* The Bhore Committee, known as the Health Survey and Development Committee, was appointed in 1943 and submitted its report in 1946. It laid emphasis on integration of curative and preventive medicine at all levels. It suggested development of one primary health centre, manned by two doctors, one nurse, four public health nurses, four midwives, four trained dais, two sanitary inspectors, two health assistants, one pharmacist, and fifteen other class IV employees, for a population of 40,000, and a secondary health centre, to provide support to PHC, and to coordinate and supervise their functioning. It also recommended major changes in medical education which includes three-month training in preventive and social medicine to prepare 'social physicians'.
- *The Mudaliar Committee (1962):* The Mudaliar Committee, headed by Dr A.L. Mudaliar, was appointed to access the performance of health sector since the submission of Bhore Committee report and it advised that the PHCs (Primary Health Centres), sub-divisional and district hospitals should be strengthened and they should provide preventive, curative, and promotive services. The Government of India appointed the Chadha Committee in 1963 to advise about the necessary arrangements for National Malaria Eradication Programme (NMEP).
- *The Chadha Committee (1963):* This committee was appointed under chairmanship of Dr M.S. Chadha, to advise about the necessary arrangements for the maintenance phase of National Malaria Eradication Programme (NMEP). The committee suggested that the vigilance activity in the NMEP should be carried out by basic health workers (one per 10,000 population), who would function as multipurpose workers and would perform, in addition to malaria work they have to perform, the duties of family planning and vital statistics data collection under supervision of family planning health assistants.

- *The Mukherjee Committee (1965):* The Government of India appointed a Mukherjee Committee headed by the secretary of health Shri Mukherjee, to review the performance in the area of family planning. The committee recommended separate staff for the family planning programme. The family planning assistants were to undertake family planning duties only. The basic health workers were to be utilized for purposes other than family planning. The committee also recommended to delink the malaria activities from family planning so that the latter would received undivided attention of its staff.
- *The Jungalwalla Committee (1967):* The Central Council of Health appointed a committee known as Committee on Integration of Health Services, in 1967, under the chairmanship of Dr N. Jungalwalla. The committee recommends integration of curative and preventive health services by the state in such a manner that the teaching and research department cadres is affected. Following steps were recommended for the integration at all levels of health organization in the country: (1) unified cadre, (2) common seniority, (3) recognition of extra qualifications, (4) equal pay for equal work, (5) special pay for special work, (6) abolition of private practice by government doctors, and (7) improvement in their service conditions.
- *The Kartar Singh Committee (1973):* This committee headed by the additional secretary of health and titled the 'Committee on multipurpose workers under health and family planning' was constituted to form a framework for integration of health and medical services at peripheral and supervisory levels. Its main recommendations were: (a) various categories of peripheral workers should be combined into a single cadre of Multi Purpose Workers (MPW) (male and female). The erstwhile auxiliary nurse midwives were to be converted into MPW (F—female) and the basic health workers, malaria surveillance workers, etc., were to be converted to MPW (M—male). The work of 3–4 male and female MPWs to be supervised by one health supervisor (male or female respectively). The existing lady health visitors were to be converted into female health supervisor;

(b) one primary health centre should cover a population of 50,000. It should be divided into 16 sub-centres (one for 3,000 to 3,500 population), etc.

- *The Srivastav Committee (1975):* This committee was set up in 1974 as 'group on medical education and support manpower' to determine steps needed to: (i) reorient medical education in accordance with national needs and priorities and (ii) develop a curriculum for health assistants who were to function as a link between medical officers and MPWs. It recommended immediate action for:
  1. Creation of bonds of para-professional and semi-professional health workers from within the community itself.
  2. Establishment of three cadres of health workers namely—multipurpose health workers and health assistants between the community level workers and doctors at PHC.
  3. Development of a 'referral services complex'.
  4. Establishment of a medical and health education commission for planning and implementing the reforms needed in health and medical education on the lines of university grants commission. Acceptance of the recommendations of the Srivastava Committee in 1977 led to the launching of the rural health service.
- *The Bajaj Committee (1986):* An expert committee for health, manpower planning, production and management was constituted in 1985 under Dr J.S. Bajaj, then the professor at All India Institute of Medical Sciences (AIIMS). Major recommendations of this committee are as follows:
  1. Formulation of national medical and health education policy.
  2. Formulation of national health manpower policy.
  3. Establishment of an Educational Commission for Health Sciences (ECHS) on the lines of UGC.
  4. Establishment of health science universities in various states and union territories.
  5. Establishment of health manpower cells at centre and in the states.

6. Vocationalization of education at 10+2 levels with regard to health-related fields with appropriate incentives, so that good quality paramedical personnel may be available in adequate numbers.
7. Carrying out a realistic health manpower survey.

Prevailing Health Structure

On the basis of the recommendation of the various committees and other national/international directives, a specific health structure has developed in India. A thorough study of the recommendations of various committees helps us to understand the growth of health services in India. The recommendations of the Bhore Committee report were never implemented in totality, although that was supposed to be the foundation stone of the development of health structure in India. The various committees responded to the specific contextual needs as identified by the government and growth of an integrated system could never become an objective. Health was never seen in a holistic perspective and the focus always remained on clinical treatment of 'diseases'. A good number of specific programmes were designed and implemented to address the specific diseases, and vertical health programmes became the core of health structure in India.

The health sector in India is characterized by: (i) a government sector that provides publicly financed and managed curative and preventive health services from primary to tertiary level, throughout the country and free of cost to the consumer (these account for about 18% of the overall health spending and 0.9 per cent of the GDP), and (ii) a fee-levying private sector that plays a dominant role in the provision of individual curative care through ambulatory services and accounts for about 82 per cent of the overall health expenditure and 4.2 per cent of the GDP. Nationwide health care utilization rates show that private health services are directed mainly at providing primary health care and financed from private resources, which could place a disproportionate burden on the poor. The provision of health care by the public sector is a responsibility shared by state, central, and local governments, although it is effectively a state responsibility in terms of service delivery (see Advani and Akram, 2007). The health care services' organization in the country extends from the national level to village level.

National and state levels: The organization at the national level consists of the Union Ministry of Health and Family Welfare. The ministry has three departments, namely, Health, Family Welfare and the Indian System of Medicine and Homeopathy (ISMH), headed by two Secretaries, one for Health and Family Welfare and the other for ISMH. The Department of Health is supported by a technical wing, the Directorate General of Health Services, headed by Director General of Health Services (DGHS). The organization at state level is under the State Department of Health and Family Welfare in each state headed by Minister and with a secretariat under the charge of Secretary/Commissioner (Health and Family Welfare) belonging to the cadre of Indian Administrative Service (IAS). By and large, the organizational structure adopted by the state is in conformity with the pattern of the central government. Every State Directorate has supportive categories comprising both technical and administrative staff. The directorate is under the charge of Director of Medical Education, who is answerable directly to the Health Secretary/Commissioner of the state. Some states have created the posts of Director (Ayurveda) and Director (Homeopathy).

Regional and district levels: In the states of Bihar, Madhya Pradesh, Uttar Pradesh, Andhra Pradesh, Karnataka, and others, zonal or regional or divisional set-ups have been created between the State Directorate of Health Services and District Health Administration. Each regional/zonal set-up covers three to five districts and acts under authority delegated by the State Directorate of Health Services. The status of officers/in-charge of such regional/zonal organizations differs, but they are known as Additional/Joint/Deputy Directors of Health Services in different states. The district-level structure of health services is a middle-level management organization and it is a link between the state as well as regional structure on one side and the peripheral-level structures such as PHC as well as sub-centre on the other side. The district officer with the overall control is designated as the Chief Medical and Health Officer (CM and HO) or as the District Medical and Health Officer (DM and HO) and is overall in-charge of the health and family welfare programmes in the district. The number of such officers, their specialization, and status in the cadre of State Civil Medical Services differ from the state to state.

Sub-divisional/taluka level: At the Taluka level, health care services are rendered through the office of Assistant District Health and Family Welfare Officer (ADHO). Some specialties are made available at the taluka hospital. The ADHO is assisted by Medical Officers of Health, Lady Medical Officers, and Medical Officers of general hospital. These hospitals are being gradually converted into Community Health Centres (CHCs).

Community level: One Community Health Centre (CHC) has been established for every 80,000 to 1, 20,000 population, and this centre provides the basic specialty services in general medicine, paediatrics, surgery, obstetrics, and gynaecology. The CHCs are established by upgrading the sub-district/taluka hospitals or some of the block-level Primary Health Centres (PHCs) or by creating a new centre wherever absolutely needed.

Primary Health Centre level: At present, there is one Primary Health Centre (PHC) covering about 30,000 (20,000 in hilly, desert, and difficult terrains) or more population. Many rural dispensaries have been upgraded to create these PHCs. Each PHC has one medical officer, two health assistants—one male and one female, and the health workers and supporting staff. For strengthening preventive and promotive aspects of health care, a post of Community Health Officer (CHO) was proposed to be provided at each new PHC, but most states did not take it up.

Sub-centre level: The most peripheral health institutional facility is the sub-centre manned by one male and one female multipurpose health worker. At present, in most places there is one sub-centre for about 5,000 populations (3,000 in hilly and desert areas and in difficult terrain).

The 73rd and 74th Constitutional Amendments have given the powers to the local bodies in some states of India. In the process, different states have adopted different stakeholders for the benefit of health services, with the help of community participation, which gives stress on safe drinking water and sanitation at village level. The panchayats are given the power to look after the welfare of the people (see, Country Health System Profile: India, Ministry of Health and Family Welfare and Health System and WHO/SEARO, for further details).

The Primary Health Centres (PHCs) and sub-centres are supposed to provide the services that cover all the essential elements of primary health care. Since 1990s, there has been a target of establishing one sub-centre staffed with health workers both female and male for a population of 5,000 in plains and 3,000 in hilly and tribal areas; and one PHC staffed with a medical officer and other paramedical staff for a population of 30,000 in plains and 20,000 in hilly and tribal areas. The number of sub-centres was 27,929 in 1971, 1,31,098 in 1991, 136,379 in 1997, and 144, 988 in 2005–06 and the number of PHCs was 725 in 1951, 5,131 in 1971, 22,243 in 1991, 22,446 in 1997, and 22,669 in 2005–06 (Kurian and Sathymala, 2008).

The secondary health care is the first referral level and the health services are generally provided by district hospitals and Community Health Centres (CHCs). The CHCs provide inpatient and outpatient services, specialist services, specialist diagnostic services, and emergency care. One CHC or an upgraded PHC with 30 beds and basic specialties is established for a population of 80,000 to 120,000 and a CHC acts as a referral centre for four PHCs. At the tertiary level, health care is provided by regional- or central-level institutions and citing WHO, Park mentions that this is more specialized than the secondary level and involves highly specialized health workers (Park, 2005). To enable the tertiary health care facilities at the regional level, Pradhan Mantri Swasthya Suraksha Yojana (PMSSY) was formulated under which six AIIMS (All India Institute of Medical Sciences) like institutions are to be set up and thirteen medical colleges are to be upgraded.

Some Health Programmes

Various vertical health programmes were launched by the Government of India (GoI) for controlling and eradicating various diseases depending upon the urgency of the situation. Presently the focus is on high morbidity due to communicable diseases, high burden of diseases due to non-communicable diseases and nutritional problems. The focus is also on the unmet need for contraception and high unwanted fertility.

The National Malaria Control Programme (NMCP) was launched by the GoI in 1953 and it was converted into National

Malaria Eradication Programme (NMEP) in 1958. In the North-eastern states (except Sikkim), selected high-risk areas of Orissa, Jharkhand, and West Bengal, an Intensified Malaria Control Project (IMCP) was implemented to make the diagnosis and treatment accessible in remote areas. National Leprosy Control Programme (NLCP) was launched by the GoI in 1955. The programme was redesigned into National Leprosy Eradication Programme (NLEP) in 1983. Further, India has the highest number of active TB cases and accounts for about one-fifth of the global TB incidence. To control TB, National Tuberculosis Control Programme (NTCP) has been in operation since 1962. The Revised National Tuberculosis Control Programme (RNTCP) was launched on 26 March 1997 with assistance from the World Bank, DFID (Department for International Development), USAID (United States Agency for International Development), GDF (Global Drug Facility), and GFATM (Global Fund for AIDS, Tuberculosis and Malaria).

The Government of India is implementing the National Iodine Deficiency Disorder Programme (NIDDCP) also, which was formerly known as National Goiter Control Programme (NGCP) since 1962. The National Cancer Control Programme was launched in 1975–76 with the aim of primary prevention, early detection, treatment, and rehabilitation. The focus of the revised programme which was completed in December 2004 is to provide cancer care facilities equally across the country. In India, several mental disorders such as schizophrenia, bipolar disorder, organic psychosis, and major depression affect nearly 20 per 1,000 population. To address the huge burden of disease, National Mental Health Programme (NMHP) was started in 1982.

The number of persons living with HIV (Human Immunodeficiency Virus) in the country is 2 to 3.1 million with an estimated adult HIV prevalence of 0.36 per cent in the country according to the revised estimates carried out during 2006. Andhra Pradesh, Karnataka, Maharashtra, and Tamil Nadu contribute 63 per cent of the HIV infected persons in the country, 39.3 per cent of infections are in women and 3.8 per cent in children. Under the National AIDS Control Programme, various steps were taken by the government: Targeted Intervention (TI) projects have been started to interrupt the transmission of HIV among highly vulnerable population which include commercial sex workers, injecting drug users, men who have sex with men, truckers, and migrant workers. The blood safety activities are an important part of National AIDS Control Programme. It is obligatory for all the blood units to get tested against the five transfusion transmissible infections (TTIs), which include HIV, Hepatitis-B, Hepatitis-C, syphilis, and malaria. Condom promotion is central to HIV/AIDS programme and during NACP-III 3.5 billion condoms are targeted to be distributed through 3 million outlets. NACO is working on a community strategy to bring about behavioural change.

Besides above-mentioned programmes, the 'kala azar' control programme was started in 1990–91 which involved providing assistance for procurement of insecticides and anti-leishmanial drugs. Kala azar is endemic in the states of Bihar, West Bengal, and parts of Uttar Pradesh. The National Health Policy, 2002 envisaged a goal of kala azar elimination by the year 2010. Further, Pulse Polio Immunization (PPI) programme was launched in 1995–96 to cover all the children below the age of three years. However, the target age group was increased from three to five years from 1996–97 to increase the speed of polio eradication.

Under the Constitution of India, public health is a shared responsibility of the central, state, and local levels of governments. However, health is essentially a state responsibility. The amount of public health spending is not uniform throughout the country but the state and local governments account for three-fourth of the total public health spending. The responsibility for the central government includes looking at port quarantine, research, and specific and technical education. On the other hand, the private health care services are provided by herbal healers, modern unqualified or quasi-qualified 'quack', and qualified practitioners of different systems of medicine. Until mid-seventies, large private hospitals were not-for-profit or charitable in nature and for-profit private hospitals were primarily small nursing homes. By 1990s, corporate sector came forward to invest in private health care and thus expanded this sector. Although most of the health care is provided by private sector, there is lack of any regulation and specification of standards for private health care. The payment in the private sector is largely fee-for-service and paid out from the pocket of the patients. There is no uniform standard for the charge of similar activities.

National Rural Health Mission (2005–12)

The Government of India, Ministry of Health and Family Welfare, launched National Rural Health Mission (NRHM) in 2005. It recognizes the importance of health as contributor of social and economic development and adopts the synergistic approach by relating health to the determinants of good health. It seeks to provide effective health care to rural population with special focus on 18 states, which have weak public health indicators. The core strategies are (a) to train and enhance capacity of Panchayati Raj Institutions (PRIs) in order to own, control, and manage public health services; (b) promote health care at household through female health activist (ASHA); (c) health plan for each village through Village Health Committee of the panchayat; (d) strengthening sub-centres through unified fund; and (f) implementation of an inter-sectoral District Health Plan. The supplementary strategies include (a) to regulate private sector including the informal rural practitioners; (b) to ensure availability of quality services to citizens at reasonable cost; (d) promotion of public-private partnerships (PPPs); (e) mainstreaming AYUSH; (f) reorienting medical education to support rural health; and (g) pooling and social health insurance to provide health security.

The NRHM has identified specific goals and objectives to be completed within a time frame. The most important initiative related to maternal health is recruitment of a new category of health worker. According to the Mission Document of NRHM, every village/large habitat will have a female Accredited Social Health Activist (ASHA)—chosen by and accountable to the panchayat—to act as the interface between the community and the public health system. ASHA would act as a bridge between the ANM and the village and be accountable to the panchayat. She will be an honorary volunteer, receiving performance-based compensation for promoting universal immunization, referral, and escort services for RCH, construction of household toilets, and other health care delivery programmes. She will be trained on a pedagogy of public health developed and mentored through a Standing Mentoring

Group at national level incorporating best practices and implemented through active involvement of community health resource organizations. She will facilitate preparation and implementation of the Village Health Plan along with Anganwadi worker, ANM, functionaries of other departments, and Self Help Group members, under the leadership of the Village Health Committee of the Panchayat. She will be promoted all over the country, with special emphasis on the 18 high focussed states. The Government of India will bear the cost of training, incentives, and medical kits. The remaining components will be funded under Financial Envelope given to the states under the programme. She will be given a drug kit containing generic AYUSH and Allopathic formulations for common ailments. The drug kit would be replenished from time to time. Induction training of ASHA will be of 23 days in all, spread over 12 months and on the job training would continue throughout the year. It also talks about prototype training material and cascade model of training proposed through 'Training of Trainers' including contract plus distance learning model. The training would require partnership with NGOs/ICDS training centres and State Health Institutes. According to a Ministry of Health and Family Welfare Report, 7.49 lakh ASHAs were selected and 7.05 lakh ASHAs were trained up to first module by 2010 (MoHFW, 2010) (see, Ministry of Health and Family Welfare, Government of India, The Journey so far 2005–10, NRHM: Meeting People's Health Needs in Partnership with States, 2010).

Janani Suraksha Yojana

Janani Suraksha Yojana (JSY) is a safe motherhood intervention under the National Rural Health Mission (NRHM) being implemented with the objective of reducing maternal and neonatal mortality by promoting institutional delivery among the poor pregnant women. The yojana, launched on 12 April 2005, is being implemented in all states and UTs with special focus on low-performing states. It is a 100 per cent centrally sponsored scheme and it integrates cash assistance with delivery and post-delivery care. The indicator of success of the scheme is the increase in institutional delivery among the poor families. The yojana has identified ASHA as an effective link between the government and the poor pregnant women in 10 low-performing states, namely the eight EAG states and Assam and Jammu and Kashmir and the remaining north-eastern states. In other eligible states and union territories, wherever, Anganwadi Worker (AWW) and Traditional Birth Attendants (TBAs) or ASHA like activist have been engaged for this purpose, she can be associated with this yojana for providing the services. The scheme focuses on the poor pregnant woman with special dispensation for states having low institutional delivery rates namely the states of Uttar Pradesh, Uttaranchal, Bihar, Jharkhand, Madhya Pradesh, Chhattisgarh, Assam, Rajasthan, Orissa, and Jammu & Kashmir. While these states have been named as low-performing states (LPS), the remaining states have been named as high-performing states (HPS). Each beneficiary registered under this yojana should have a JSY. ASHA/AWW/any other identified link worker under the overall supervision of the ANM, the MO, and PHC should mandatorily prepare a micro-birth plan. This will effectively help in monitoring antenatal check-up, and the post-delivery care. Under this programme, the delivering mother and the recommending ASHA from rural areas will get cash assistance of ₹ 1,400 and ₹ 600, respectively, after the first and second institutional delivery. The amount for the urban areas is ₹ 1,000 and ₹ 200, respectively.

Rashtriya Swasthya Bima Yojana (RSBY)

RSBY has been launched by Ministry of Labour and Employment, Government of India, from 1 April 2008 to provide health insurance coverage for below poverty line (BPL) families. The objective of RSBY is to provide protection to BPL households from financial liabilities arising out of health shocks that involve hospitalization. Beneficiaries under RSBY are entitled to hospitalization coverage up to ₹ 30,000 for most of the diseases that require hospitalization. The government has even fixed the package rates for the hospitals for a large number of interventions. Pre-existing conditions are covered from day one and there is no age limit. Coverage extends to five members of the family, which includes the head of household, spouse, and up to three dependents. Beneficiaries need to pay only ₹ 30 as registration fee while central and state governments pay the premium to the insurer selected by the state government on the basis of a competitive bidding (see Government of India website, http://www.rsby.gov.in/ about_rsby.html).

References

Advani, M. and Akram, M. (2007). 'Health Concerns in India', in M. Akram (ed.), *Health Dynamics and Marginalised Communities* (pp. 3–26), Jaipur: Rawat Publications.

Akram, M. (2012a). 'Challenges Before Health Planning in India: Preparing Draft of the 12th Five-year Plan', *Journal of US-China Public Administration*, 9(2): 229–234.

Bagchi, A.K. and Soman, K. (2005). *Maladies, Preventives and Curatives, Debates in Public Health in India*, New Delhi: Tulika Books.

Country Health System Profile: India, Ministry of Health and Family Welfare and Health System. Ministry of Health and Family Welfare, Government of India, official website.

Kurian, N.J. and Sathymala, C. (2008). 'Health Sector in India: Issues and Challenges' in *India Social Development Report: Development and Displacement*, New Delhi: Oxford University Press

Ministry of Health and Family Welfare, Government of India, (2010) The Journey so far 2005–10, NRHM: Meeting People's Health Needs in Partnership with States, 2010.

Qadeer, I. (1985). 'Health Service System in India: An Expression of Socio-Economic Inequalities' *Social Action*, 35.

WHO. (1952). *Report of Expert Committee on Public Health Administration*,

WHO/SEARO. http://www.rsby.gov.in/about_rsby.html

Chapter Fifteen

Health Policies and Planning in India

India had its first National Health Policy (NHP) in 1983 and before it only vertical health programmes such as National Malaria Control Programme (NMCP), National Leprosy Eradication Programme, National Tuberculosis Control Programme, National Cancer Control Programme, etc., existed, which were meant to address specific diseases (discussed elsewhere in this book). The first National Health Policy tried to revamp public health sector and specified the target of health for all by 2000 as its specific goal. Before presenting the summary of the 1983 policy, it is important to know the background under which this policy came into existence. The background is related to the Alma Ata Declaration. The International Conference on Primary Health Care, held at Alma Ata, USSR, 6–12 September 1978, has conceived the vision of 'Health for All'. Globally, it was decided that every state must target to achieve the goal of health for all by 2000. This declaration has given direction to the health policy and planning of national governments, all over the world.

Declaration of Alma Ata

The International Conference on Primary Health Care, meeting in Alma Ata this twelfth day of September in the year nineteen hundred and seventy-eight, expressing the need for urgent action by all governments, all health and development workers, and the world community to protect and promote the health of all the people of the world, hereby makes the following declaration:

(i) The Conference strongly reaffirms that health, which is a state of complete physical, mental, and social well-being, and not merely the absence of disease or infirmity, is a fundamental human right and that the attainment of the highest possible level of health is a most important world-wide social goal whose realization requires the action of many other social and economic sectors in addition to the health sector.

(ii) The existing gross inequality in the health status of the people particularly between developed and developing countries as well as within countries is politically, socially, and economically unacceptable and is, therefore, of common concern to all countries.

(iii) Economic and social development, based on a New International Economic Order, is of basic importance to the fullest attainment of health for all and to the reduction of the gap between the health status of the developing and developed countries. The promotion and protection of the health of the people is essential to sustained economic and social development and contributes to a better quality of life and to world peace.

(iv) The people have the right and duty to participate individually and collectively in the planning and implementation of their health care.

(v) Governments have a responsibility for the health of their people which can be fulfilled only by the provision of adequate health and social measures. A main social target of governments, international organizations, and the whole world community in the coming decades should be the attainment by all peoples of the world by the year 2000, a level of health that will permit them to lead a socially and economically productive life. Primary health care is the key to attaining this target as part of development in the spirit of social justice.

(vi) Primary health care is an essential health care based on practical, scientifically sound, and socially acceptable methods and technology, made universally accessible to individuals and families in the community through their full participation and at a cost that the community and country can afford to maintain at every stage of their development in the spirit of self-reliance and self-determination. It forms an integral part both of the country's health system, of which it is the central function and main focus, and of the overall social and economic development of the community. It is the first level of contact of individuals, the family, and community with the national health system bringing health care as close as possible to where people live and work, and constitutes the first element of a continuing health care process.

(vii) Primary health care:

1. reflects and evolves from the economic conditions and socio-cultural and political characteristics of the country and its communities and is based on the application of the relevant results of social, biomedical and health services research, and public health experience;
2. addresses the main health problems in the community, providing promotive, preventive, curative, and rehabilitative services accordingly;
3. includes at least education concerning prevailing health problems and the methods of preventing and controlling them; promotion of food supply and proper nutrition; an adequate supply of safe water and basic sanitation; maternal and child health care, including family planning; immunization against the major infectious diseases; prevention and control of locally endemic diseases; appropriate treatment of common diseases and injuries; and provision of essential drugs;
4. involves, in addition to the health sector, all related sectors and aspects of national and community development, in particular agriculture, animal husbandry, food, industry, education, housing, public works, communications, and other sectors; and demands the coordinated efforts of all those sectors;
5. requires and promotes maximum community and individual self-reliance and participation in the planning,

organization, operation, and control of primary health care, making fullest use of local, national, and other available resources; and to this end develops through appropriate education the ability of communities to participate;

6. should be sustained by integrated, functional, and mutually supportive referral systems, leading to the progressive improvement of comprehensive health care for all, and giving priority to those most in need;
7. relies, at local and referral levels, on health workers, including physicians, nurses, midwives, auxiliaries, and community workers as applicable, as well as traditional practitioners as needed, suitably trained socially and technically to work as a health team and to respond to the expressed health needs of the community.

(viii) All governments should formulate national policies, strategies, and plans of action to launch and sustain primary health care as part of a comprehensive national health system and in coordination with other sectors. To this end, it will be necessary to exercise political will, to mobilize the country's resources, and to use available external resources rationally.

(ix) All countries should cooperate in a spirit of partnership and service to ensure primary health care for all people since the attainment of health by people in any one country directly concerns and benefits every other country. In this context, the joint WHO/UNICEF report on primary health care constitutes a solid basis for the further development and operation of primary health care throughout the world.

(x) An acceptable level of health for all the people of the world by the year 2000 can be attained through a fuller and better use of the world's resources, a considerable part of which is now spent on armaments and military conflicts. A genuine policy of independence, peace, détente, and disarmament could and should release additional resources that could well be devoted to peaceful aims and in particular to the acceleration of social and economic development of which primary health care, as an essential part, should be allotted its proper share.

•

The International Conference on Primary Health Care calls for urgent and effective national and international action to develop and implement primary health care throughout the world and particularly in developing countries in a spirit of technical cooperation and in keeping with a New International Economic Order. It urges governments, WHO and UNICEF, and other international organizations, as well as multilateral and bilateral agencies, non-governmental organizations, funding agencies, all health workers, and the whole world community to support national and international commitment to primary health care and to channel increased technical and financial support to it, particularly in developing countries. The Conference calls on all the aforementioned to collaborate in introducing, developing, and maintaining primary health care in accordance with the spirit and content of this declaration.

National Health Policy, 1983

The main focus of the National Health Policy (NHP), adopted in 1983, was the formulation of an integrated and comprehensive approach towards future development of health services, appropriately supported by medical education and research, with special emphasis on PHC and related support services. During the Seventh Five-Year Plan, there was considerable achievement in terms of establishment of a health infrastructure, especially in rural areas. The Eighth Plan (1992–97) identified 'human development' as its main focus, with health and population control listed as two of six priority objectives. It was emphasized that health facilities must reach the entire population by the end of the eighth plan. The plan also identified peoples' initiative and participation as a key element. With the enactment of the 73rd Constitutional Amendment Act (1992), PRIs were revitalized and a process of democratic decentralization ushered in, with similar provisions made for urban local bodies, municipalities, and nagar palikas.

Recognizing the importance of sustainable development, a national conservation strategy and a policy statement on environment and development were formulated in 1992 to bring environmental considerations into the developmental process. Linkages were drawn between poverty, population growth, and the environment. The NHP identified nutrition as a problem needing urgent attention and in 1993 a National Nutrition Policy was formulated with long- and short-term strategies.

The vertically structured family welfare programme needed to be replaced by a more democratic, decentralized alternative. In 1994, a draft national population policy was submitted to parliament as well as a revised report in 1996. It advocated a holistic, multisectoral approach towards population stabilization, with no targets for specific contraceptive methods except for achieving a national average Total Fertility Rate (TFR) of 2.1 by the year 2010. This has resulted in a radical shift in implementation from centrally fixed targets to a target-free dispensation through a decentralized, participatory approach. A Population and Social Development Commission was also established in support of the population policy.

India has accepted the recommendations of the ICPD (1994) and has also ratified various international conventions for securing equal rights for women. Following the World Summit on Survival, Protection and Development of Children in 1990, India formulated a Plan of Action for Children in 1992 with actions that directly and indirectly affect child health.

While overall mortality has declined considerably, living standards are still among the poorest in the world. The major constraints facing the health sector are lack of resources, lack of an integrated support, poor involvement of NGOs, inadequate laboratory services, poor disease surveillance and response systems, and the heavy investments needed in dealing with non-communicable diseases. The problems of gender disparity still manifest themselves in various forms, as evidenced by the declining female to male population ratio, social stereotyping, violence at the domestic and social level, and continuing open discrimination against the girl child, adolescent girls, and women.

Thus, the period after the last National Health Plan was announced in 1983 has seen major developments in India. There has been an increase in mortality through 'lifestyle' diseases—diabetes, cancer, and cardiovascular diseases. The increase in life expectancy has increased the requirement for geriatric care. Similarly, the increasing burden of trauma cases is also a significant public health problem. The changed circumstances relating to the health sector of the country since 1983 have generated a situation in which the government has undertaken steps to formulate a new policy framework as the National Health Policy, 2002. But the government failed in realizing the objectively defined targets of health and had to shift its priorities and directions under the structural adjustment programme (SAP) of 1990s.

The decade of 1990s, known for several economic and structural reforms and moving towards liberalization, privatization, and globalization (LPG), resulted in important shifts even in the health policy. Three important things noticed then were: (1) increasing participation of voluntary organizations and private corporations; (2) increasing the quality of care at tertiary level; and (3) user charges even at the public health care centres. Further, just at the turn of the century and arrival of the new millennium, the world got a new vision, in terms of the Millennium Development Goals (MDGs). Just as the Alma Ata Declaration was thrust behind the NHP, 1983, the MDGs became the thrust for the NHP, 2002. We will discuss the salient features of both here.

Millennium Development Goals (MDGs)

Millennium Development Goals (MDGs) are the specific goals of social transformation designed for the entire world at the beginning of the 21st century. MDGs are a set of numerical and time-bound targets to measure achievements in human and social development. The MDGs originated from the Millennium Declaration produced by the United Nations. The Millennium Declaration outlined the most ambitious global agenda till date for eradicating poverty and preventable disease, promoting equitable development, and protecting the earth's environment. The Declaration asserts that every individual has the right to dignity, freedom, equality, a basic standard of living that includes freedom from hunger, disease, and violence, and encourages tolerance and solidarity. The MDGs were made to operationalize these ideas by setting targets and indicators for poverty reduction and health improvement.

The MDGs are eight international development goals that all 192 member states of United Nations and at least 23 international organizations have agreed to achieve by the year 2015. The eight goals are eradicate extreme poverty and hunger, achieve universal primary education, promote gender equality and empower women, reduce child mortality rates, improve maternal health, combat HIV/AIDS, malaria, and other diseases, ensure environmental sustainability, and develop a global partnership for development. All these goals are directly or indirectly related to improvement in health status of individuals and communities. Major successes in combating extreme poverty, improving school enrolment and child health, and controlling spread of killer deceases such as AIDS, Malaria, and TB in almost all developing countries—even in the poorest countries—demonstrate that the Millennium Development Goals (MDGs) are achievable (MDG-ICR, 2011).

The MDGs do not say everything that needs to be said about health and development. They say nothing about the importance of effective health systems which are essential to the achievement of all health goals, about reproductive health or non-communicable diseases. We therefore have to understand the MDGs as a form of shorthand for some of the most important outcomes that development should achieve. The health-specific goals of MDGs resulted in: fewer women dying in childbirth; more children surviving the early years of life; dealing with the catastrophe of HIV/AIDS; making sure people have access to life-saving drugs; and better health—in all its forms—making a major contribution to the reduction of poverty.

National Health Policy (2002)

The second National Health Policy (NHP, 2002) came in the aftermath of Millennium Development Goals (MDGs) (as discussed above). The NHP, 2002 is a revised and much improved version of the NHP of 1983 and it has incorporated many of the health-related goals and objectives suggested by the MDGs. The NHP, 2002 prescribed the following measures: (1) to increase the health sector expenditure to 6 per cent of GDP (Gross Domestic Product), with 2 per cent of GDP being contributed as public health investment, by the year of 2010; (2) to reduce the various kinds of inequities and imbalances; (3) to increase allocation of 55 per cent of the total health investment for the primary health sector, 35 per cent and 10 per cent for secondary and tertiary sectors respectively;

(4) great emphasis to be laid down upon the implementation of public health programmes through local self-government institutions; (5) need for specialists in public health and family medicine; (6) need for an improvement in the ratio of nurses vis-à-vis doctors/beds; (7) welcoming private sector in all areas of health activities; (8) emphasis on the need for simplifying the procedures for government civil society interfacing to enhance the involvement of civil society in public health programmes; and (9) need for providing secondary and tertiary health service, to users from overseas who have the ability to pay. However, it could not succeed in achieving the 'objectively' defined goals because of several reasons, and lack of funds and poor infrastructure were important among them (for details, see policy document National Health Policy, 2002, available at Government of India website).

Universal Health Coverage (UHC)

An important development, after the MDGs, at the global level, related to health policy and planning, is the development of a new vision of Universal Health Coverage (UHC) for citizens at national level. Member-states of the WHO committed in 2005 to develop their health financing systems so that all people have access to services and do not suffer financial hardship paying for them. This goal was defined as universal coverage, sometimes called universal health coverage. Across the world, more than 100 million people are pushed into poverty each year because of health care expenditures. This is an avoidable tragedy. Striving for the goals of universal accessibility and affordability of health and health care, WHO proposed a model for Health Systems Financing (WHO, 2010). This report and the suggested roadmaps are going to have important implications in health policy and planning in India. The Government of India constituted a High Level Expert Group (HLEG) in 2010(HLEG, 2011) for suggesting the model of Universal Health Coverage (UHC) for India. It had six terms of references (ToRs). Out of these, the most important are related to financing; resource generation; ensuring access to essential drugs, vaccines and medical technology; and allowing participation of private for-profit sectors in delivery of health care in India. However, the ToRs ignored an important component that WHO had suggested: an equitable coverage and not an equal coverage to all. An equitable coverage is the best possible means to address the problems of health inequality that India is increasingly realizing. On the insistence of some of the members, a ToR related to social determinants of health coverage has also been included in the report submitted by the HLEG.

The World Health Report (WHO, 2010), suggesting roadmaps for health systems financing and universal coverage, is a lengthy report. The 'Message from the Director-General' of WHO gives the vision of the report. It is reproduced here for understanding the core thrust of the report:

> I commissioned this world health report in response to a need, expressed by rich and poor countries alike, for practical guidance on ways to finance health care. The objective was to transform the evidence, gathered from studies in a diversity of settings, into a menu of options for raising sufficient resources and removing financial barriers to access, especially for the poor. As indicated by the subtitle, the emphasis is firmly placed on moving towards universal coverage, a goal currently at the centre of debates about health service provision.
>
> The need for guidance in this area has become all the more pressing at a time characterized by both economic downturn and rising health care costs, as populations age, chronic diseases increase, and new and more expensive treatments become available. As this report rightly notes, growing public demand for access to high-quality, affordable care further increases the political pressure to make wise policy choices.
>
> At a time when money is tight, my advice to countries is this: before looking for places to cut spending on health care, look first for opportunities to improve efficiency. All health systems, everywhere, could make better use of resources, whether through better procurement practices, broader use of generic products, better incentives for providers, or streamlined financing and administrative procedures.
>
> This report estimates that from 20 per cent to 40 per cent of all health spending is currently wasted through inefficiency and points to 10 specific areas where better policies and practices could increase the impact of expenditures, sometimes

dramatically. Investing these resources more wisely can help countries move much closer to universal coverage without increasing spending.

Concerning the path to universal coverage, the report identifies continued reliance on direct payments, including user fees, as by far the greatest obstacle to progress. Abundant evidence shows that raising funds through required prepayment is the most efficient and equitable base for increasing population coverage. In effect, such mechanisms mean that the rich subsidize the poor, and the healthy subsidize the sick. Experience shows this approach works best when prepayment comes from a large number of people, with subsequent pooling of funds to cover everyone's health care costs.

No one in need of health care, whether curative or preventive, should risk financial ruin as a result.

As the evidence shows, countries do need stable and sufficient funds for health, but national wealth is not a prerequisite for moving closer to universal coverage. Countries with similar levels of health expenditure achieve strikingly different health outcomes from their investments. Policy decisions help explain much of this difference.

At the same time, no single mix of policy options will work well in every setting. As the report cautions, any effective strategy for health financing needs to be home-grown. Health systems are complex adaptive systems, and their different components can interact in unexpected ways. By covering failures and setbacks as well as successes, the report helps countries anticipate unwelcome surprises and avoid them. Trade-offs are inevitable, and decisions will need to strike the right balance between the proportion of the population covered, the range of services included, and the costs to be covered.

Yet despite these and other warnings, the overarching message is one of optimism. All countries, at all stages of development, can take immediate steps to move towards universal coverage and to maintain their achievements. Countries that adopt the right policies can achieve vastly improved service coverage and protection against financial risk for any given level of expenditure. It is my sincere wish that the practical experiences and advice set out in this report will guide policy makers in the right direction.

> Striving for universal coverage is an admirable goal, and a feasible one—everywhere (Dr Margaret Chan, Director-General, World Health Organization).

Time will tell the larger implication of the model provided by WHO and achievements made by the national government in India in ensuring the goal of health for all.

References

Alma Ata Declaration. (1978) Available online at: http://www.who.int/social_determinants/tools/multimedia/alma_ata/en/ (accessed 6 October 2011).

HLEG (2011)., High Level Expert Group Report on Universal Health Coverage for India: Instituted by Planning Commission of India. Available online at: http://planningcommission.nic.in/reports/genrep/rep_uhc0812.pdf (accessed 5 July 2012).

Millennium Development Goals (MDGs). Available online at www.un.org/millenniumgoals/ (accessed 6 October 2011)

Millennium Development Goals: India Country Report. Available online at: http://www.undp.org/content/india/en/home/library/mdg/mdg_india_country_report_2011.html. (accessed 10 May 2012).

National Health Policy. (2002). Ministry of Health and Family Welfare, Government of India 2002. Available online at: http://www.mohfw.nic.in/NRHM/Documents/National_Health_policy_2002.pdf (accessed 8 March 2012).

National Rural Health Mission. (2005). Available online at: accessed 5 July 2012). http://www.mohfw.nic.in/NRHM/Documents/NRHM_Framework_Latest.pdf (accessed 8 March 2012)

WHO. (2005). 'Sustainable Health Financing, Universal Coverage and Social Health Insurance', in *Fifty-eighth World Health Assembly*, Resolution WHA58.33. 16–25 May 2005. Geneva, WHO. Available online at: http://apps.who.int/gb/ebwha/pdf_files/WHA58–REC1/english/A58_2005_REC1–en.pdf (accessed 23 June 2010).

WHO. (2010). *The World Health Report: Health Systems Financing: The Path to Universal Coverage*. Available online at: www.who.int/entity/whr/2010/overview.pdf (accessed 5 July 2012).

CHAPTER SIXTEEN

Inequality, Inequity, and Dehealthism in Health

Indian society is characterized by multiple inequalities. Whereas caste and gender divides find their roots in socio-historical complexes, class and spatial divides are related to uneven politico-economic developments. Cutting across these structural inequalities, 'health inequality' is a more contemporary consequence of poor investment on public health, improper development planning, and narrow health policy designs. India is witnessing differential achievements in increasing the life expectancy at birth and controlling infant mortality, maternal mortality, and long- and short-term communicable and non-communicable morbidities among and within various states and social categories. The increasing hiatus in health achievements among groups in India amidst growing medicalization and other reforms suggest prevalence of a deeper creeping malaise: health inequality. Health inequality, according to Amartya Sen, is one of the basic forms of inequality.

The Alma Ata Declaration made in 1978 (see previous chapter) stated that 'attainment of the highest possible level of health is a most important world-wide social goal whose realization requires the action of many other social and economic sectors in addition to the health sector'. It further says that 'the existing gross inequality in the health status of the people particularly between developed and developing countries as well as within countries is politically, socially, and economically unacceptable and is, therefore, of common concern to all countries'. The Alma Ata Declaration and many other studies carried out in the last two decades of the twentieth century exposed the widespread inequalities inherent in the health condition of the people. The inequalities in health reveal not only the inequalities present in various other segments of the society but also a result of various ongoing social, cultural, and politico-economic processes. Cross-national evidences suggest that the greater the degree of socio-economic inequality exits within a society, the steeper the gradient of health inequality.

In the words of Daniels, Kennedy, and Kawachi (2006: 63), '... middle-income groups in a more unequal society will have worse health than comparable or even poorer groups in a society with greater equality'. Health inequality is not always the result of economic inequality. In the words of Michael Marmot (2006: 38), '... wider inequalities in health represent wider inequalities in society—although the evidence on this is still problematic'. However, differences in health among individuals in society are different from inequalities between social groups. Our concern here is mainly with group inequalities and not individual differences within the groups (see Akram and Beg, in press).

'Why' and 'How' of Inequality in Health

According to Amartya Sen, health contributes to a person's basic capability to function. Hence, health is the most basic requirement for every individual. Denial of health is not only denial of 'good life-chance'; it is also denial of fairness and justice. Sen has helped to make the capabilities approach a paradigm for policy debate in human development where it inspired the creation of the UN's Human Development Index. Alkire (2003) has explained the capability approach through its four main components:

- *Functionings:* Sen regards functionings as doings and beings which create a better conceptual space to examine social welfare than utility or opulence. The focus of capability approach on functionings takes the capability approach away from other approaches used to evaluate well-being. Alkire gives an example of how in economic theory welfare is interpreted in term of psychological happiness and desire fulfilment, but magnitude of change in mental utility states may not predict the value of change. Sen often quote an example of how the deprived become compatible with their circumstances and appreciate small mercies, thus their desires are muted and their psychological pleasure at small improvements to their situation is not proportionate to the benefit judged from another perspective. Sen questions Rawl's proposal to require equality in the space of primary goods and argues that Rawl's reasoning can be broadened to take greater note of the contingency of circumstances.

- *Freedom:* Capability refers to the freedom of persons or groups to promote or achieve things which they consider valuable and it was used by Sen to attend to the foundational importance of freedom.
- *Pluralism:* Sen emphatically defends the breadth of the capability approach and the pluralism of its information base. Sen argues that individual advantage can be examined in four different spaces which include well-being achievement, well-being freedom, agency achievement, and agency freedom. Sen also argues that we cannot focus on any one of these four possible spaces and that these may be in conflict with each other. Capability approach widens the information basis of considerations than inform the social welfare and social choice analysis and thus in this way it supports the pluralism.
- *Incompleteness:* Incompleteness is one of the most important advantages of capability approach and for allowing incompleteness; Sen identifies two grounds—fundamental and pragmatic. The capability approach of Sen is intentionally incomplete and the reason behind this is to allow economists and development practitioners to work on pressing issues for which consensus on fundamentals is not required.

The roots of capability approach go back to Adam Smith, Karl Marx, and Aristotle. Sen argues that these functionings have to be examined and the capability of a person to achieve them has to be valued appropriately. The functionings may vary from primary functionings such as avoiding morbidity and mortality to many complex functionings such as achieving self-respect (Sen, 2006b). Robeyns (2006) argues that the difference between a functioning and a capability is the same as the difference between an achievement and the freedom to achieve something and between an opportunity and an outcome. All capabilities correspond to the overall freedom to lead a life that one has reason to value. Sen criticizes the theories that focus extensively on utility resource or income but Sen does not deny the important contribution resources can make to peoples well-being as inequalities in resources can indeed be an important cause of inequalities of capabilities (see, Beg, 2011).

The capability approach, according to Peter (2006), provides a useful alternative for accessing health problems in society. Good health is often regarded by Sen as an example of functioning (e.g., as used by Sen in his 'Capability and Freedom'). Peter, however, points out that it is more favourable to use health as a capability or a subset of capability because of the fact that health itself is composed of various functionings such as ability to move around, not being tired and others. Sen leaves it open that which functionings are to be included while accessing a particular social situation. Sen stresses that in each case, this will require a process of selecting a relevant functioning and weighing their relative importance. Seeing health as a capability or a subset of capability requires a process that involve value judgements and which is subjected to political contestation. Thus, the process of defining health and determining what counts as health and what as another type of social problems cannot be solved by the health specialists alone but depends on other aspects of social institutions, and may change over time.

Health inequality does not mean any kind of health difference (or biological differences) but the differences in health which are potentially avoidable. Inequality in health can be explained as a particular type of difference in health that could be potentially shaped by policies. It is a difference in which disadvantaged social groups (such as poor, racial/ethnic minorities, women, or other groups that have persistently experienced social disadvantage or discrimination) systematically experience worse health or greater health risks than more advantaged social groups. Health inequalities or disparities include comparison not only between the best- and worst-off groups in a given category (e.g., the richest versus the poorest), but between the most socially disadvantaged groups and all others (Heggenhougen and Quati, 2008).

Anand (2006) has argued that there should be more aversion to inequalities in health than inequalities in income because health has both instrumental and intrinsic value, while income has only instrumental value. Inequalities in health are closely related to inequalities in the most basic freedom and opportunities that people can enjoy. Some income inequalities are justified because, as often asserted by economists, income incentives are required to elicit effort, skill, enterprise, and so on. These incentives or difference in reward increase the size of total income from which the society as a whole can gain. This increase has to be balanced against the income inequalities that must be tolerated in order to provide appropriate incentives for efficiency. In addition to this effort, skill, enterprise, and so on are regarded as, are considered as, fair and legitimate means for some people to earn. But inequalities in health constitute inequalities in the capability of people to function. The investigation of health inequalities between groups helps to find out the groups that suffer from poor health and are at high risk, so that these might be targeted directly for the improvement in health and it helps to bring forth health inequalities which are regarded as unfair and unjust.

The Black Report (1980) is a landmark document in health inequality research, which brought about a paradigm shift in the discourse of health inequalities. Though it was well known that poorer sections of a community are more prone to disease and death but there were debates among the various groups regarding the cause. The hereditarians believed that people's social position was determined by inherent natural abilities, the public health doctors believed that the material conditions of poor led to the debilitating health, independent of inherited constitutions, and another stream which later congeal into behavioural school of public health believed that unhealthy and reckless behaviour on the part of the poor was responsible for their poor health. The Black Report pointed out the complex effects of the economy and different forms of social organization, including the family, upon the level of health.

While studying the patterns of morbidity, mortality, and utilization of health services across different occupational group in Britain, the Black Report brought to light marked inequality between the various classes on the basis of occupation for both the sexes and for all the ages. It also pointed out those inequalities in health continued to increase in spite of the growth in economy in England. According to Mukopadhyay (2008), the Black Report provided four possible explanations for these inequalities: (i) artefact explanation, according to which the changes were because of the statistical problems; (ii) the natural and social selection approach according to which the people who are healthy are able to move higher on the social ladder; (iii) material and social selection approach, which gave importance to role of economic deprivation; and (iv) the cultural explanation, which primarily focus on individual behaviour, ideas, and motivation. The report argues that although various sets of explanations are needed over time to clearly understand the inequalities in health, the materialist explanation is consistent of all the four.

The general finding that prosperity and health are related give an impression that income/health gradient are unavoidable. Daniels, Kennedy, and Kawachi (2006) using data of United Nations Human Development Report Statistics come to the conclusion that there is a clear relation between GDP (Gross Domestic Product) per capita and life expectancy, which is clearer in advanced industrial economies, but this relationship exist up to a certain level. They also pointed out that relationship between health and income is not fixed, and the nation's health achievement is mediated by processes other than wealth. Various other factors such as culture, social organization, and policies of government are also the determinants of health, and the variation in these factors also explains the difference in health outcome. Thus, if health of nations reflects policy choices or the features of the society that can be changed through policies, then we must ask about the justice or injustice of alternate policies.

The Foucauldian approach towards health and disease can also be applied to understand the health inequalities. Michel

Foucault calls attention to an important aspect of modern society: it is an administered society, in which professional groups define categories of people—the sick, the insane, the criminal, the deviant—on behalf of an administrative state. For Foucault, medicine is a product of the administrative state, policing normal behaviour, and using credentialed professionals to enforce compliance with the 'normal'. Thus, health inequalities are also a product of the administrative state and its governmentality. In the democratic governments and welfare economies, government play most important role in policy making and deciding administrative priorities. Hence, a critical analysis of the government policies and planning designs is very important towards understanding the perpetual causation of health inequalities in modern societies.

Health Inequity in India

According to the Planning Commission document 'An Approach to the Twelfth Five-Year Plan' (2011), the total expenditure on health in India in the Eleventh Plan, as a percentage of GDP, was around 5 per cent (which is roughly comparable to other developing countries). However, within this, there was a disproportionally high reliance on private, particularly household's out-of-pocket expenditure. This reflected a critical imbalance in the health care system, which stemmed from deficiencies in the public sector's capacity to deliver basic health care. The private sector too was characterized by wide variations. At one end of the spectrum were private hospitals with world-class facilities and personnel offering services, which were competitively priced compared to similar services abroad, but remained beyond the capacity of most Indians. At the other end, there was an unregulated private sector which was more affordable, but offered services of varying quality, often by under-qualified practitioners.

Further, the Ministry of Health and Family Welfare document, 'Annual Report to the People on Health' (MoHFW, 2010) states that from a public policy point of view, it is desirable that health financing is so arranged that it reduces the overall out-of-pocket (OoP) expenditure on health care, and protects against financial catastrophe related to health care. The global standard related to the 'desirable' limit of OoP to protect people from financial catastrophe is less than 15 per cent of total health spending. In contrast, in India, the OoP is to the tune of 71 per cent of total health spending. It is also important to note here that the per capita public health spending is low in India, being among the five lowest in the world. The public health expenditure in the country over the years has been comparatively low, and as a percentage of GDP it has declined from 1.3 per cent in 1990 to 0.9 per cent in 1999, increased marginally to 1.1 per cent by 2009. The Central budgetary allocation for health over this period, as a percentage of the total central budget, has been stagnant at 1.3 per cent, but has almost doubled to 2 per cent by 2008–09. Taking cognisance of the important role of public health expenditure, the Eleventh Five-Year Plan (2007–12) document suggests the necessity of building a responsive public health system with the need for increasing the public spending on health from 0.9 per cent of GDP to 2–3 per cent of GDP and stepping up investment on primary care, communicable diseases, and HIV/AIDS prevention.

Further, the public spending on health accounts for around 1 per cent of the GDP. This ratio is among the lowest in the world, although in recent years the share of public spending in total health spending has been steadily increasing. An important issue in public spending on health relates to the distribution between the central and state sectors. With the launch of National Rural Health Programme (NRHM), the level of public spending on health has risen nearly 2.6 times between 2004–05 and 2009–10 (the estimates for 2009–10 are budget estimates). The share of the central government in the total health expenditure (including grants-in-aid to states through treasury and society routes) increased from 32.1 per cent in 2004–05 to 38.4 per cent in 2007–08.

Out-of-pocket expenditure (OoP) on health care forms a major barrier to health seeking in India. According to the National Sample Survey Organization (NSSO), the year 2004 saw 28 per cent of ailments in rural areas go untreated due to financial reasons—up from 15 per cent in 1995–96. Similarly, in urban areas, 20 per cent of ailments were untreated due to financial reasons—up from 10 per cent in 1995–96. Those who access 'free' government health services are expected to purchase medicines from private pharmacies, pay user fees for laboratory tests and of course the ubiquitous informal fees. Those who use the private services of course have to pay considerable amounts. Significantly, those who are insured also do not get full protection. While their OoP payments are reduced, they still have to pay for ambulatory care and for excluded conditions. It is clear that Indians (especially the vulnerable sections) do not have any form of financial protection and are forced to make OoP payments when they fall sick. This is regressive and has both economic and social consequences (Annual Report to the People on Health, 2010).

Across the world, more than 100 million people are pushed into poverty each year because of health care expenditures. This is an avoidable tragedy. Responding to the initiative of WHO to find new means and ways for coverage of health needs of people, Government of India constituted a High Level Expert Group (HLEG) in 2011 for suggesting a new model of Universal Health Coverage (UHC), for providing universal accessibility and affordability of health care for all Indians. The HLEG has made several observations. It reports that, in a rapidly globalizing world, millions continue to experience profound inequities in health, living, working, and too often, dying in conditions of poverty, exclusion, and disenfranchisement. The greatest successes of health system reform—be it primary health care in Cuba, the right to health paradigm of Brazil, or abolishing out-of-pocket spending in Thailand—have addressed the wider determinants of health inequities as a national priority, implementing reform through both policy changes and grassroots-based action. India is marked by disparities in both exposure and vulnerability to diseases and access to health services, with the poorest and most disadvantaged being most affected. The latter include urban and rural poor, women, children, specially abled persons, and the traditionally marginalized and excluded groups such as adivasis, scheduled tribes (STs), dalits, scheduled castes (SCs) as well as ethnic and religious minorities.

The HLEG suggests that more than a fourth of the world's population who are hungry are Indians. As per the WHO's standards, 40 per cent of Indian children under the age of three are underweight, 45 per cent are stunted, and 23 per cent have wasting. Talking about the situation of water and sanitation, it reports a study of urban poor communities in Mumbai which found that water-related illnesses accounted for almost a third of all morbidity in the last year among adults, and almost two-thirds of all morbidity among children. Another study in five Indian states found a negative correlation between the provision of household toilets and community-level prevalence of communicable diseases including cholera, typhoid/enteric disease, diarrhoea/vomiting, hepatitis, nematodal infections as well as malaria and dengue. A 2002 Planning Commission report expressed alarm over the 'rather extensive presence' of fluoride and arsenic in Indian drinking water, which is associated with a number of cancers (of the skin, lungs, kidneys, and bladder). Further, provisional data from the 2011 Census suggests that gender inequity is a persistent and worsening phenomenon in India, occurring throughout the life cycle: a 13 point decline in the male-female sex ratio from 927 females per 1,000 males in 2001 to 914 females per 1,000 males in 2011 suggests that as more families are having fewer children, gendering of sex composition is rising.

Developing Indicators of Health Inequality and Inequity

Inequality is both subjective and objective. Economic inequalities can be measured quantitatively. But inequality in status is often a subjective phenomenon. Inequality in health is both subjective and objective. The capability approach makes a contemporary effort to understand the causes as well as possible consequences of inequalities in health. The biomedical approach towards health and disease explains some inequalities in health attainment as biological or genetic differences. However, the social determinant approach says that even the biological or genetic factors are socially caused. Hence, Sen and many other prefer the term inequity over inequality to explain the differential achievement in health attainment. Inequities in health are avoidable and can be corrected through proper policies and implementation. Foucauldian approach, which talks about the role of administration and governance and discourses of power, is relevant here. However, there is increasing effort by social scientists to explain the inequalities and inequities on the basis of some objectively identifiable indicators.

Life Expectancy

In terms of life expectancy, child survival, and maternal mortality, India's performance has improved steadily. However, there are wide divergences in the achievements across the states. There are inequities based on rural-urban divides, gender imbalances, and caste patterns. Life expectancy in India has more than doubled in the last 60 years. It increased from around 30 years at the time of independence to over 63.5 years in 2002–06. But the wide variance in performance across states is of special concern. While in Kerala, a person at the time of birth is expected to live for 74 years, the expectancy of life at birth in states such as Assam, Bihar, Madhya Pradesh, Orissa, Rajasthan, and Uttar Pradesh is in the range of 58–62 years, a level Kerala achieved during the period 1970–75. Globally, India's life expectancy is lower than the global average of 67.5 years.

Infant Mortality Rate (IMR)

India's infant mortality rate (IMR) too has shown a steady decline, from 129 deaths per 1,000 live births in 1971 to 53 in 2008. The rate of decline has been slowing, from 19 points in the 1970s to 16 points in the current decade. The disparity between urban and rural is very high as urban IMR is 36 as compared to the rural IMR of 58. Widespread disparities are also visible among various social categories in India. The IMR per 1,000 live births among scheduled castes (SCs), scheduled tribes (STs), other backward classes (OBCs), and others is 66.4, 62.1, 56.6 and 57 respectively. The highest per cent of underweight children (under 5 years age) is among SCs (54.5) and lowest is among others (33.7). The other disparities or differential outcome among the high- and low-performing states is given in Table 1.

The MMR estimates of Bihar, Madhya Pradesh, and Uttar Pradesh also apply to Jharkhand, Chhattisgarh, and Uttarakhand respectively (as compiled by Annual Report to the People on Health, MoHFW, 2010).

Table 1 Key demographic health indicators

High Focus States EAG	*Life Expectancy at Birth (2002–06)*	*IMR (2008)*	*MMR (2004–06)*	*TFR (2008)*
1	*2*	*3*	*4*	*5*
Bihar	61.6	56	312	3.9
Madhya Pradesh	58.0	70	335	3.3
Orissa	59.6	69	303	2.4
Rajasthan	62.0	63	388	3.3
Uttar Pradesh	60.0	67	440	3.8
Assam	—	64	480	2.6
Kerala	74.0	12	95	1.7
Maharashtra	67.2	33	130	2.0
Punjab	69.4	41	192	1.9
Tamil Nadu	66.2	31	111	1.7
West Bengal	64.9	35	141	1.9
INDIA	63.5	53	254	2.6

Note: IMR: Infant Mortality Rate, MMR: Maternal Mortality Ratio, TFR: Total Fertility Rate, '—': Not available

Source: (col. 2) to Col. (4): Registrar General of India; Planning Commission.

Maternal Mortality Ratio (MMR)

Maternal health is a key indicator of women's health and status. Maternal Mortality Ratio (MMR) measures the number of women aged 15–49 years dying due to maternal causes per 1,00,000 live births. India had a MMR of 460 in 1984, which declined to 254 deaths per 1,00,000 live births in 2004–06. Great disparity is visible among the states even in MMR as Kerala and Tamil Nadu report low MMR of 95 and 111 respectively, whereas other states have high MMR, namely, Assam (480), Bihar/Jharkhand (312), Madhya Pradesh/Chhattisgarh (335), Orissa (303), Rajasthan (388), and Uttar Pradesh/Uttarakhand (440) (MoHFW, 2010).

Maternal Care

Antenatal care (ANC) refers to pregnancy-related health care, which is usually provided by a doctor or health professional. The main purposes of antenatal care are to prevent certain complications, such as anaemia, and identify women with established pregnancy complications for treatment or transfer. According to NFHS–3, almost one out of every five women in India did not receive any antenatal care for their last birth in the 5 years preceding the survey. Women not receiving antenatal care tend disproportionately to be older women, women having children of higher birth orders, scheduled tribe women, women with no education, and women in households with a low wealth index. The utilization of antenatal care services differed greatly by state; Kerala and Tamil Nadu each ranked highest on four of the nine indicators but Arunachal Pradesh, Nagaland, Uttar Pradesh, Jharkhand, and Rajasthan performed poorly on most of the indicators. Compared with Tamil Nadu, for example, where 96 per cent of mothers had three or more antenatal care visits, only 17 per cent of mothers in Bihar and 27 per cent in Uttar Pradesh had three or more visits.

For India, as a whole, mothers of only 15 per cent of births received all of the required components of antenatal care. This indicator ranges from a high of 64 per cent in Kerala and 56 per cent in Goa to a low of only 2 per cent in Nagaland and 4 per cent in Uttar Pradesh. Other states that performed almost as poorly as Uttar Pradesh and Nagaland on this indicator included Bihar, Arunachal Pradesh, Madhya Pradesh, Jharkhand, Meghalaya, Rajasthan, and Mizoram, where only 6–9 per cent of women received the recommended components of antenatal care. Kerala, followed closely by Goa, also outperformed all other states in terms of delivery care, with nearly all deliveries taking place in medical institutions and a similarly high percentage of deliveries assisted by a health professional. By contrast, only 12–20 per cent of births were delivered in medical institutions in Nagaland, Chhattisgarh, Jharkhand, and Bihar. Only 25–29 per cent of deliveries are assisted by health professionals in Nagaland, Uttar Pradesh, Jharkhand, and Bihar (NFHS–3).

Communicable and Non-communicable Diseases

According to WHO, over 5.2 million people died in India of non-communicable diseases (NCDs) such as cardiovascular diseases, stroke, diabetes, and cancer in 2008. NCDs accounted for

53 per cent of all deaths. Among men, 38 per cent of the deaths were under 60 years, while among women it was 32 per cent. Cardiovascular diseases accounted for 24 per cent of all deaths, cancers (6%), respiratory disease (11%), diabetes (2%), and other NCDs (10%). NCDs are the top cause of death worldwide, killing more than 36 million in 2008. Cardiovascular diseases were responsible for 48 per cent of these deaths, cancers (21%), chronic respiratory diseases (12%), and diabetes (3%). One of the findings shows that men and women in low-income countries are around three times more likely to die of NCDs before 60 years than in high-income countries. These differential outcomes in health indicators are obvious indication of perpetuating health inequalities (Sinha, 2011; WHO, 2011).

Types of Disparities in Health

Both inequalities and inequities are disparities. Ali and Nanda (2006) have argued that four forms of inequalities can be identified in the field of health. The various kinds of health disparities inherent in India are briefly discussed here:

- *Geographic disparities:* Fertility rates are not uniform among the states. Only two of the fifteen major states have reached the replacement level of fertility, that is, 2.1. Another five major states have total fertility rate of between 2.1 and 3, and in the eight major states (comprising about 44% of population) the rate is 3 or more. Infant mortality, maternal mortality, and expected life at birth also vary significantly among various states and often within the states. These differences are largely because of poverty, illiteracy, and inadequate access to health care facilities and family welfare services.
- *Gender disparity:* In India, the disparities in health on the basis of gender are particularly prominent. The largest gender disparities are found in the northern states, particularly Haryana and Punjab despite their relative prosperity. Girls have low mortality rates than boys during the first month of life (the neonatal period) which accounts for their lower rate of infant mortality. However, cited by Indian Institute of Population Studies, death rates in the postneonatal and in the whole period up to five years of age (under-5 mortality) are

higher for girls as compared to boys. Despite having lower rates of acute respiratory infections, diarrhoea, and anaemia, which are major causes of childhood death, boys as compared to girls continue to have higher rates of mortality. This paradox exists because of the fact that boys are more likely to receive health care than girls and also the girls have higher rates of malnutrition which places them at further disadvantage. The relative neglect of women's health is also depicted in the poor reproductive health indicators.

- *Disparity among Scheduled Tribes and Scheduled Castes:* Of all the disadvantaged groups in India, SCs tend to have the highest rates of infant and child mortality, malnutrition, and morbidity followed by SCs and then by other disadvantaged (or backward) classes.
- *Poverty disparity:* Communicable diseases, malnutrition, and maternal conditions are concentrated among the poor in India. The rich people are less sick, become sick at an old age and suffer more from non-communicable diseases than from the communicable diseases in comparison to poorer population. Levels of mortality, morbidity, and malnutrition are higher among the poor than among the rich. The poorest quintile has double the risk of infant and child deaths, malnutrition, and high fertility in comparison to the richest quintile.

What Can Be Done?

Disparities in health can be removed. Amarjeet Sinha, in Annexure 2 of the report of the HLEG, gives evidences from global communities. According to Sinha, there is an evidence of reduction in undernutrition over a short period of time. A few examples are as follows:

- In People's Republic of China, life expectancy increased from 35 years to 67 years and IMR dropped from 200 to 42, between 1949 and 1979. This happened on account of five very basic measures—food security, clean water and sanitation, basic public health measures, a barefoot doctor in every village, and full immunization. Between 1990 and 2002, child malnutrition reduced by more than half, from 25 per cent to 8 per cent.

- Thailand halved child malnutrition from 50 per cent to 25 per cent between 1982 and 1986 through a network of Community Health Volunteers.
- Vietnam reduced malnutrition from 45 per cent to 27 per cent between 1990 and 2006.
- Brazil reduced child malnutrition from 18 per cent to 7 per cent between 1975 and 1989. During the same period, IMR came down from 85 to 36.

Sinha has identified the common factors behind success. The success in the countries listed above is attributable, in most cases, to very basic interventions—Community Health Worker, food security, guaranteed clean water, sanitation thrust, focus on behaviour change communication, full immunization, basic public health measures, and a functional primary health care system. The HLEG also talks about the increasing departmentalism within the government and ministries, as an important reason of lack of coordination at the policy and planning level.

A Critical Analysis

The health policy in India is heavily dominated by the biomedical approach. The government is focused on developing infrastructure for clinical treatment of diseases assuming that diseases are ubiquitous and inevitable. However, the ecological and socio-cultural approaches suggest that diseases are preventable and health is not just absence of diseases but much more than that. Health is directly related to food, nutrition, potable water, healthy and hygienic environment, proper living conditions, affordable and accessible health care facilities, and an equitable, accountable, and just delivery mechanism.

Identifying some of the continuities and gaps in the existing health policy and planning in India (as discussed in previous chapters), this author claims that health inequality in India, to a great extent, is a consequence of cumulative wrongs at the level of policy prioritization and planning. This author gives an integrated analysis with new conceptual terms and formulations. It revisits the Alma Ata Declaration (1978) which states that primary health care includes at least: (i) education concerning prevailing health problems and the methods of preventing and controlling them; (ii) promotion of food supply and proper nutrition; (iii) an adequate supply of safe water and basic sanitation; (iv) maternal and child health care, including family planning; (v) immunization against the major infectious disease; (vi) prevention and control of locally endemic disease; (vii) appropriate treatment of common disease and injuries; and (viii) provision of essential drugs. Out of these eight primary elements necessary for primary health care, this author considers unadulterated nutritious food, safe drinking water, and sanitation as the 'Basic Health Goods (BHGs)'. Health for all is just an illusion without the comprehensive presence of the BHGs in any society but more particularly in developing societies like India.

Empirical data as discussed above suggest that many of the states in India have lackadaisical approach towards making universal availability of BHGs. The practice of denying BHGs to the population or a part of it or even gradual withdrawal from it is denial of health chance and can conveniently be termed as 'dehealthism'. Any group, community, or state practising dehealthism can't achieve the goal of health for all, no matter how much medicalization it is promoting. It is important to note here that increasing medicalization of the health structures has created several discourses surrounding health, some of which are: primary health, basic health, holistic health, curative health, preventive health, promotive health, rehabilitative health, public health, and community health. All these variants of health are meaningless if the concerned group is a victim of dehealthism.

Dehealthism is also related to the notion of medicalism. Medicalism promotes medicalization in several senses: identifying new medical territories, increasing medical hegemony and gaze, pharmaceuticising the food and drinks, etc., are some of the popular forms (as discussed in the chapter on Medicalization and Demedicalization). One of the consequences of medicalism, in India, is narrowing the field of 'primary health care'. The notion of primary health centre (the most important functional unit of health structure) in India is much narrower than what is prescribed in the Alma Ata Declaration and says nothing about the BHGs. One further variant of medicalism in India is capturing the budgetary allocations for health (The NRHM scams is a great testimony). The last two consequences of medicalism are related to dehealthism. Narrowing the scope or budget of primary health and exclusion of BHGs is also dehealthism. However, dehealthism is much more than it.

Some of the states in India are increasingly withdrawing from its responsibilities of providing public health (under the cumulative influence of globalization, privatization, and pauperization). This is again dehealthism. There is a new proposed modality of universal health coverage which suggests policies such as mediclaims and medicares for reimbursing the medical care cost of individuals and groups. Such coverage of the expenditure made on treatment of disease often covers the interest of private health care provider as well as the insurance companies. However, when such coverage is promoted as substitutes of primary health care provided by the state, it is dehealthism. Dehealthism reduces the territory of holistic health and perpetuates the conditions responsible for causation of disease and illness and attracts medical interventions and medicalization. Health inequality in India is a result of the medical hegemony, invisible networking of vested interests (INVIs), and a vicious circle of medicalism and dehealthism.

Empirical studies conducted at various levels suggest significant relationship between health achievement of the population and levels of income and educational attainment. But, the India Human Development Report, 2011 suggests that the improvement in the Health Index during the period 1999–2000 to 2007–08 is well below the improvement in the Human Development Index (HDI) overall. It reflects that, while the Income Index has improved at the same rate as the HDI for India, and the Education Index by much more than the improvement in the HDI, the Health Index has not shown any significant change. Thus, correlations between health and education or income cannot necessarily lead us to the argument that removal of income and educational inequality is the precondition for removal of health inequality (and will automatically reduce health inequalities). The social determinant of health hypothesis (which finds its efficacy in western industrial and developed societies) is often selectively and discriminatorily used to support the arguments that health inequalities are simply the consequences of prevailing income and educational inequalities. Keeping in mind the poor performance of various states in India in removing poverty or attaining universal primary education, removal of health disparity will become a distant dream if we continue to believe in the above causation. Treating health as completely dependent variable on income, education, and lifestyle/chances legitimizes the dismal performance of the health care agencies and arbitrarily decided non-coherent health policy priorities in many of the states.

The author suggests that a mere increase in budgetary allocation or privatization or even public-private partnership is not a panacea for achieving the desired health goals and combating the deep malaise of health inequality in India. Health should be seen from a comprehensive perspective and should not be seen from only biomedical perspective. Public health policy should be revived. Along with focussing on medicine and curative health, all the basic health goods should also be made available and accessible to the most needful. The increasing medicalization of health needs, and especially the basic health goods, should be stopped. Preventive and community health should be promoted as per the guideline of Alma Ata Declaration. The vested interest, involved at various levels should be identified and exposed and the unseen constraints should be properly addressed. And last but not the least, a better coordination among all the agencies be developed so that a better communication and reciprocation with the stake holders can be achieved. Health allocation must be increased (up to 5% of GDP) and a separate budget (2% of GDP) be allocated for providing BHGs and combating dehealthism in India.

Some of the arguments and texts in this chapter is included from a research paper entitled 'Looking Beyond the Universal Health Coverage: Health Inequality, Medicalization and Dehealthism in India' sent for publication in a refereed international journal, *Public Health Research*. The paper is not published and hence due reference or acknowledgement cannot be made at this stage. However, the arguments are important for the potential readers of the book and the acknowledgement is necessary for the potential publisher of the paper.

References

Akram, M. and Beg, S.R. (in press). 'Health Inequalities in India and the Challenges before Social Transformation', in Modi, I. (ed.), *Polity, Civil Society, Development and Agrarian Issues: Essays honouring Professor Yogendra Singh*, Jaipur: Rawat Publications.

Ali, A. and Nanda, A.R. (2006). 'Health Sector: Issues and Challenges', in *India Social Development Report 2006*, New Delhi: Oxford University Press.

Alkire, S. (2003). *Valuing Freedoms: Sen's Capability Approach and Poverty Reduction*, New Delhi: Oxford University Press.

Anand, S. (2006). 'The Concern for Equity in Health', in Anand, S., Peter, F., and Sen, A. (eds.), *Public Health, Ethics and Equity* (pp. 15–20), New Delhi: Oxford University Press.

Beg, S.R. (2011). *Health Inequities in India: A Review of Literature* (Unpublished M. Phil. Dissertation), Maulana Azad Central Library, AMU, Aligarh.

Black Report. (1980). *Inequalities in Health: Report of a Research Working Group*, DHSS.

Foucault, M. (1973). *The Birth of Clinic*, First published by Tavistock Publications Limited in 1973, First published in Routledge Classics in 2003, Oxon.

Heggenhougen, H.K. and Quati, S.R. (2008). *International Encyclopaedia of Public Health*, Vol. 3 J-O, USA: Elsevier Academic Press.

Marmot, M. (2006). 'Social Causes of Social Inequalities in Health', in Anand, S., Peter, F., and Sen, A. (eds.), *Public Health, Ethics and Equity*, New Delhi: Oxford University Press.

MoHFW (Ministry of Health and Family Welfare). (2010). *Annual Report to the People on Health*, New Delhi: Government of India.

Mukopadhyay, I. (2008). 'Analysing Health Inequalities: Social Capital and Its Infirmities', *Social Scientist*, Vol. 36: 11–12.

Peter, F. (2006). 'Health Equity and Social Justice', in Anand, S., Peter, F. and Sen, A. (eds.), *Public Health, Ethics and Equity*, New Delhi: Oxford University Press.

Planning Commission. (2011). *Report of the Working Group on Disease Burden for the 12th Five-Year Plan: WG-3 (1): Communicable Diseases*, No. 2 (6) 2010.

Robeyns, I. (2006). 'Sen's Capability Approach and Gender Inequality: Selecting Relevant Capabilities', in Agarwal, B., Humphires, J. and Robeyns, I. (eds.), *Capability, Freedom and Equality: Amartya Sen's Work from a Gender Perspective*, New Delhi: Oxford University Press.

Sen, A. (2006b). 'Development as Capability Expansion', in Agarwal, B., Humphires, J., and Robeyns, I. (eds.), *Capability, Freedom and Equality: Amartya Sen's Work from a Gender Perspective*, New Delhi: Oxford University Press.

World Health Organization. (2011). *Non-communicable Diseases Country Profiles 2011*. Available online at: http://whqlibdoc.who.int/publications/2011/9789241502283_eng.pdf. (accessed 8 March 2012).

Bibliography

Advani, M. (1980). *Doctor-Patient Relationship in Indian Hospitals*, Jaipur: Sanghi Prakashan.

Advani, M. and Akram, M. (2007). 'Health Concerns in India', in M. Akram (ed.), *Health Dynamics and Marginalised Communities* (pp. 3–26), Jaipur: Rawat Publications.

Aggarwal, A.K., Kumar, R. and Gupta, V. et al. (1999). 'Community-based Study of Reproductive Tract Infections among Ever Married Women of Reproductive Age in a Rural Area of Haryana, India', *Journal of Communicable Diseases*, 31(4): 223–228.

Aggleton, P. (1990). *Health*, London: Routledge Publications.

Agrawal, K.G. and Advani, M. (1972). 'Development of a Model for Ward Social System', *Interdiscipline*, 9: 29–39.

Akram, M. (2005a). 'STDs and the Tribal Population', *Indian Journal of Sexually Transmitted Diseases*, 26(1): 17–22.

——. (2005b). 'Sustainable Development, Health and STDs: A Study of Tribal Society of Rajasthan', *Social Change*, 35(3): 99–110.

——. (2008). *Tribal Health: Studying Sexual Behaviour*. Jaipur: Rawat Publications.

——. (2012a). 'Challenges Before Health Planning in India: Preparing Draft of the 12th Five-year Plan', *Journal of US-China Public Administration*, 9(2): 229–234.

——. (2012b). 'Development of Sociology of Health: A Review of the Contexts and Phases, Themes and Future in India', *Salute e Società (Sociology and sociology of health: A round trip)*,, XI-2 (English) 89–115.

——. (ed.). (2007). *Health Dynamics and Marginalized Communities*, Jaipur: Rawat Publications.

Akram, M. and Beg, S.R. (in press). 'Health Inequalities in India and the Challenges Before Social Transformation', in Modi, I. (ed.), *Polity, Civil Society, Development and Agrarian Issues: Essays Honouring Professor Yogendra Singh*, Jaipur: Rawat Publications.

Ali, A. and Nanda, A.R. (2006). 'Health Sector: Issues and Challenges', in *India Social Development Report 2006*, New Delhi: Oxford University Press.

Alkire, S. (2003). *Valuing Freedoms: Sen's Capability Approach and Poverty Reduction*, New Delhi: Oxford University Press.

Anand, S. (2006). 'Concern for Equity in Health', in Anand, S., Peter, F. and Sen, A. (eds.), *Public Health, Ethics and Equity*, New Delhi: Oxford University Press, 15–20.

Andersen, M.L. and Taylor, H.F. (2011). *Sociology: The Essentials*, sixth edition, USA: Wadsworth, Cengage Learning.

Awasthi, S. and Pande, V.K. (1998). 'Sexual Behaviour Patterns and Knowledge of Sexually Transmitted Diseases in Adolescent Boys in Urban Slums of Lucknow', *Indian Paediatrics*, 35(11): 1105–1109.

Baer, H., Singer, M. and Johnsen, J. (1986). 'Towards a Critical Medical Anthropology', *Social Science and Medicine*, 23: 95–98.

Bagchi, A.K. and Soman, K. (2005). *Maladies, Preventives and Curatives, Debates in Public Health in India*, New Delhi: Tulika Books.

Bajpai, N. and Dholakia, R.H. (2011). *Improving the Integration of Health and Nutrition Sectors in India*, Columbia Global Centres/South Asia, Columbia University.

Bakhru, H.K. (2010). *A Complete Handbook of Nature Cure.* Mumbai: Jaico Publishing.

Banerji, D. (1971). 'Tuberculosis: A Problem of Social Planning in India', *NIHAE Bulletin*, IV (1): 9–25.

——. (1974). 'Social and Cultural Foundations of the Health Services Systems of India', *Economic and Political Weekly*, 9 (32–34): 1333–1346.

——. (1982). *Poverty, Class and Health Culture in India*, Vol. I, New Delhi: Prachi Prakashan.

——. (1985). *Health and Family Planning Services in India*, New Delhi: Lok Paksh.

——. (2001). 'Landmark in the Development of Health Services in India', in Qadeer, I. Sen, K. and Nayar, K.R. (eds.), *Public Health and the Poverty of Reforms* (pp. 37–38), New Delhi: Sage Publications.

Banerji, D. and Anderson, S. (1963). 'A Sociological Study of Awareness of Symptoms among Persons with Pulmonary Tuberculosis', *Bulletin of the WHO*, 29(5): 665–683.

Bardhan, A., Sinha, S.K., Gopinath, K., et al. (1989). *A Study of Factors Responsible for Less or No Utilization of Health Facilities among the Bhils of Madhya Pradesh.* PAC Report (Mimeo), New Delhi: NIHFW.

Barry, A.M. and Yuill, C. (2002). *Understanding Health: A Sociological Introduction*, London/Thousand Oaks/New Delhi: Sage Publications.

Baru, R.V. (1993). 'Inter-regional Variations in Health Services in Andhra Pradesh', *Economic and Political Weekly*, 28(20): 963–967.

——. (1998). *Private Health Care in India: Social Characteristics and Trends*, New Delhi: Sage Publications.

Baru, R.V., Qadeer, I. and Priya, R. (2001). 'State and Private Sector in India: Some Policy Options', in Nandraj, S., Muraleedharan, V.R., Baru, R.V., et al. (eds.), *Private Health Sector in India: Review and Annotated Bibliography* (pp. 51–71), Mumbai: CEHAT.

Barua, A. and Kurz, K. (2001). 'Reproductive Health-seeking by Married Adolescent Girls in Maharashtra, India' *Reproductive Health Matters*, 9(17): 53–62.

Basu, D.P. (1994). 'Appropriate Methodologies for Studying Sexual Behaviour in India', *Indian Journal of Social Work*, LV(4): 573–588.

Basu, S. and Mitra, K. (2001). 'Health Development of Tribal Communities of India: Need for Action Research', *Indian Journal of Social Development*, 1(1): 134–156.

Basu, S.K. (1986). 'Genetics, Socio-cultural and Health Care among Tribal Groups of Jagdalpur and Konta Tehsils of Bastar District, M.P.', in A.K. Kalla and K.S. Singh (eds.), *Anthropology, Development and Nation Building* (pp. 87–105), New Delhi: Concept Publishing Company.

——. (1994). 'A Health Profile of Tribal India', *Health Millions*, 2(2): 12–14.

——. (1995). 'Health Status of Tribal Woman in India', in Singh, B. and Mohanty, N. (eds.), *Tribal Health in India* (pp. 57–92), New Delhi: Inter-India Publications.

Beg, S.R. (2011). *Health Inequities in India: A Review of Literature*, Unpublished M. Phil. Dissertation, Maulana Azad Central Library, AMU, Aligarh.

Bhandari, B. (1989). *Tribal Marriages and Sex Relations*, Udaipur: Himanshu Publication.

Bhardwaj, R. (2010). 'Medical Pluralism in India: The Interface of Complementary and Alternative Therapies with Allopathy', in Mishra, A. (ed.), *Health, Illness and Medicine: Ethnographic Readings*, New Delhi: Orient Blackswan.

Bhasin, V. (2007). *Medical Anthropology: A Review*, Delhi: Department of Anthropology, University of Delhi.

Bhatia, A.K. (1967). 'Needs and Problems of Patients', *Nursing Journal of India*, 48(5): 210–212.

Bhatia, J.C. and Cleland, J. (2001). 'Health Care Seeking and Expenditure by Young Indian Mothers in the Public and Private Sectors', *Health Policy and Planning*, 16(1): 55–61.

Bhatia, R. (1992). 'Socio-economic Inequalities and Health Status', *Economic and Political Weekly*, XXVII(51–52): 2702–2703.

——. (2007). 'Health Policy, Plan and Implementation: The Role of Health Workers in Altering the Sex Ratio', in Patel, T. (ed.), *Sex Selective Abortion in India: Gender, Society and New Reproductive Technologies* (pp. 203–231), New Delhi: Sage Publications.

Bhattacharjee, J., Gupta, R.S. and Kumar, A., et al. (2000). 'Pre- and Extra-marital Heterosexual Behaviour of an Urban Community in Rajasthan', *Journal of Communicable Diseases*, 32(1): 33–39.

Bhende, A.A. (1994). 'A Study of Sexuality of Adolescent Girls and Boys in Underprivileged Groups in Bombay', *Indian Journal of Social Work*, LV(4): 557–571.

Black Report. (1980). *Inequalities in Health: Report of a Research Working Group*, DHSS.

Bonita, R., Beaglehole, R. and Kjellström, T. (2006). *Basic Epidemiology*, second edition, Geneva: World Health Organization.

Borins, M. (1987). 'Traditional Medicine in India'. Can. Fam. Physician, April. vol. 33, Available online at http://www.ncbi.nlm.nih.gov/pmc/articles/PMC2218447/

Bose, A. (1982). 'Health Policy in India: 1947–81', in K. D Madan, et al., (eds.), *Policy Making in Government Publication Division* (pp. 501–519), New Delhi: Government of India.

Bose, A. and Desai, P.B. (1983). *Studies in Social Dynamics of Primary Health Care*, Delhi: Hindustan Publishing House.

Brym, R.J. and Lie, J. (2007). *Sociology: Your Compass for a New World*, third edition, United Kingdom: Thomson Wadsworth.

Calnan, M. (1987). *Health and Illness: The Lay Perspective*, London: Tavistock.

Cant, S. and Sharma, U. (1999). *A New Medical Pluralism*, London/New York: Routledge Publications.

Carstairs, G.M. (1955). 'Medicine and Faith in Rural Rajasthan', in Paul, B.D. (ed.), *Health, Culture and Community* (pp. 107–134), New York: Russel Sage Foundation.

Chandani, A. (1985). *The Medical Profession: A Sociological Exploration*, New Delhi: Jainsons.

Chatterjee, S.C. (2010). 'Intervertebral Disc Prolapse: A Personal Encounter with Biomedicine', in Mishra, A. (ed.), *Health, Illness and Medicine: Ethnographic Readings* (pp. 61–74), New Delhi: Orient Blackswan.

Chatterjee, S.C. and Roy, T. (2005). 'Coping with Genetic Disorder: A Sociological Understanding of Parent Caregivers' Experiences', *Illness Crises and Loss*, 13(4): 315–331.

Chaudhury, S.K. (2006). *Culture, Ecology and Sustainable Development*, New Delhi: Mittal Publications.

——. (2006). *Thinkers and Theories in Sociology: From Comte to Giddens*, Delhi: Gangandeep Publications.

Chowdhary, P.D. (1977). *Concept of Disease and Methodology of Treatment (Medical and Non-medical) in West Bengal* (Unpublished Ph.D. Thesis), Calcutta University.

Clarke, J. (1981). 'A Multiple Paradigm Approach to the Sociology of Medicine, Health and Illness', *Sociology of Health and Illness*, 3(1): 89–103.

Cockerham, W.C. (2001). *Medical Sociology*, Upper Saddle River, NJ. Prentice Hall.

——. (2007). *Social Causes of Illness and Disease*, USA: Polity Publication.

——. (2010). *Medical Sociology*, Oxford, UK: Blackwell.

——. (2010). *The Blackwell Companion to Medical Sociology*, Oxford, UK: Blackwell Publishers.

Cockerham, W.C. and Ritchey, F.J. (1997). *Dictionary of Medical Sociology*, London: Greenwood Press.

Coe, R.M. (1970). *Sociology of Medicine*, New York/London: McGraw-Hill Book Company.

Conant, J. (2005). *Sanitation and Cleanliness for a Healthy Environment*, Hesperian Foundation, USA.

Conrad, P. (1975). 'The Discovery of Hyperkinesis: Notes on the Medicalization of Deviant Behaviour', *Social Problems*, 23.

——. (2007). *The Medicalization of Society: On the Transformation of Human Conditions into Treatable Disorders*, Baltimore, Maryland: Johns Hopkins University Press.

Conrad, Peter and Schneider, J.W. (1980). *Deviance and Medicalization: From Badness to Sickness*. Michigan: Mosby

Country Health System Profile: India, Ministry of Health and Family Welfare and Health System.

Dak, T.M. (1991). *Sociology of Health in India*, Jaipur: Rawat Publications.

Darulius, Z. and Kaminskas, R. (2007). *Peculiarities of Medical Sociology: Application of Social Theories in Analyzing Health and Medicine*, Lithuiania: Kunas University of Medicine.

Das, V., Das, R.K. and Coutinho, L. (2000). 'Disease Control and Immunization: A Sociological Enquiry', *Economic and Political Weekly*, 35(8–9): 625–632.

David, B. (1987). 'The Value of Labour-Power and Health', in Scambler, G. (ed.), *Sociological Theory and Medical Sociology*, London: Tavistock; McKinley.

De Maio, F. (2010). *Health and Social Theory*, New York: Palgrave Macmillan.

Dingwall, R. (1976). *Aspects of Illness*, London: Martin Robertson.

Djurfeldt, G. and Lindberg, S. (1976). *Pills Against Poverty: A Study of the Introduction of Western Medicine in a Tamil Village*, New Delhi: Oxford and IBH Publishing Company.

Dubey, S.C. (1971). *Cultural Factors in Health: A Case Study from Madhya Pradesh—A Project Report*. Sagar: Department of Anthropology and Sociology.

Elwin, V. (1955). *The Religion of an Indian Tribe*, London: Oxford University Press.

Environment, Water and Sanitation, Irish Aid Key Sheet, Environment Policy for Sustainable Development, www.irishaid.gov.ie.

Environmental Health in India: Priorities in Andhra Pradesh. (2001). Environment and Social Development Unit South Asia Region, October.

Epidemiology and Surveillance. (2006). Treguine Refugee Camp, Chad, November, The Johns Hopkins and the International Federation of Red Cross and Red Crescent Societies.

Epidemiology Program Office. (n.d.). *Principles of Epidemiology; An Introduction to Applied Epidemiology and Biostatistics*, second edition, US Department of Health and Human services, Public Health Service, Centres for Disease Control and Prevention, Epidemiology Program Office, Atlanta, Georgia.

Foucault, M. (1973). *The Birth of Clinic*, Tavistock Publications. First published by Tavistock Publications Limited in 1973, First published in Routledge Classics in 2003, Oxon.

Gabe, J., Bury, M. and Elson, M. (2004). *Key Concepts in Medical Sociology*, London: Sage Publications.

Ganatra, B.R. and Hirve, S.S. (2002). 'Induced Abortions among Adolescent Women in Maharashtra, India', *Reproductive Health Matters*, 10(19): 76–85.

Gandhi, A., Kumar, C., Saha, P., Kishore, B., et al. (2011). *India Human Development Report; Towards Social Inclusion*, Institute of Applied Manpower Research, Planning commission, Government of India, Oxford University Press, New Delhi.

Gangadharan, G.G. and Shankar, D. (2009). 'Medical Pluralism: The Challenges Ahead', *Indian Journal of Traditional Knowledge*, 8(2): 181.

Gangolli, L.V., Duggal, R., and Shukla, A. (2005). *Review of Healthcare in India*, Mumbai: Centre for Enquiry into Health and Allied Themes, Research Centre of Anusandhan Trust, Survey No. 2804 and 2805.

Gerhardt, U. (1989). *Ideas about Illness: An Intellectual and Political History of Medical Sociology*, Basingstoke: Macmillan.

Giddens, A. (2006). *Sociology*, fifth edition, Cambridge: Polity Press.

Giri, T.K., Wali, J.P., Meena, H.S., et al. (1995). 'Socio-demographic Characteristics of HIV Infection in Northern India', *Journal of Communicable Diseases*, 27(1): 1–9.

Global Hunger Index: The Challenge of Hunger: Focus on the Crisis of Child Undernutrition. (2010). International Food Policy Research Institute, Concern Worldwide and Welthungerhilfe. Available online at: www.ifpri.org/publication/2010–global-hunger-index

Goffman, E. (1961). *Asylums*, New York: Doubleday and Anchor.

Gould, H.A. (1965). 'Modern Medicine and Folk Cognition in Rural India', *Human Organization*, 24(3): 201–208.

Graham, H. (1993). *When Life's a Drag: Women, Smoking and Disadvantage*. London: HMSO

Guidotti, T. (ed.). (2011). *Global Occupational Health*, New York/New Delhi: Oxford University Press.

Hang, Y. (2008). *Encyclopaedia of Global Health*, London/New Delhi: Sage Publications.

Hansen, E. and Easthop, G. (2007). *Lifestyle in Medicine*, London/New York: Routledge, Taylor and Francis Group.

Harshal T.P. (2008). 'Environmental Sanitation: An Ignored Issue in India'

Hasan, K.A. (1967). *The Cultural Frontier of Health in Village India*. Bombay: Manaktalas.

——. (1980). *Medical Sociology of Rural India*, Ajmer: Sachin Publications.

Health System in India: Crisis and Alternatives', 2006, National Health Assembly II Booklet 2 by National Coordination Committee, Jan Swasthya Abhiyan.

Heggenhougen, H.K., Quati, S.R. (2008). *International Encyclopaedia of Public Health*, Vol. 3 J-O, USA: Elsevier Academic Press.

HLEG. (2011). Report of the High Level Expert Group on Universal Health Coverage, Planning Commission, Government of India. Available online at: http://planningcommission.nic.in/reports/genrep/rep_uhc0812.pdf.

Hobson, W. (ed.). (1965). *The Theory and Practice of Public Health*, New York: York: Oxford University Press.

Jayaram, N. (1977). 'Social Implications of Medical Education in India', *Journal of Higher Education*, Autumn: 207–220.

Jeffery, R. (1978). 'Allopath Medicine in India: A Case of Deprofessionalisation', *Economic and Political Weekly*, 13(3): 101–113.

Jefferys, M. (1969). 'Sociology and Medicine: Separation or Symbiosis', *Lancet*,1(7606): 1112–1116.

Jenkins, C.D. (2003). *Building Better Health: A Handbook of Behavioural Change*, Scientific and Technical Publication No. 590, Pan American Sanitary Bureau, Washington, DC.

Jesani, A. and Iyer, A. (1993). 'Women and Abortion', *Economic and Political Weekly*, 28(48): 2591–2594.

Kakar, D.N., Srinivas Murthy, S.K. and Parker, R.L. (1972). 'People's Perception of Illness and Their Use of Medical Care Services in Punjab', *Indian Journal of Medical Education*, XI: 286–298.

Kanbargi, R. and Kanbargi, S. (1996). 'STDs in Bangalore City: Some Findings from an Exploratory Study', *The Journal of Family Welfare*, 42(1): 30–37.

Karuna, C. (2001). 'Hinduism and Female Sexuality: Social Control and Education of girls in India', *Sociological Bulletin*, 50(1): 37–63.

Kaur, M. (1991). 'Maternity and Child Health: A Socio-cultural Analysis', in Dak, T.M. (ed.), *Sociology of Health in India* (pp. 217–229), Jaipur: Rawat Publications.

Kelman, S. (1975). 'The Social Nature of the Definition Problem in Health', *International Journal of Health Services*, 5: 625–642.

Kendall, D. (2011). *Sociology in Our Times*, eighth edition, CA,USA: Wadsworth, Cengage Learning.

Khan, S. (1994). 'Cultural Contexts of Sexual Behaviour and Identities and Their Impact Upon Preventive Models: An Overview of South Asian Men Who Have Sex with Men', *Indian Journal of Social Work*, 55(4): 633–646.

Kleinman, A. (1988). *The Illness Narratives: Suffering, Healing and the Human Condition*, New York: Basic Books.

Knox, D. (2008). *Understanding Social Problem*, USA: Wordsworth Cengage.

Kumar, G.S., Kar, S.S. and Jain, A. (2011). 'Health and Environmental Sanitation in India: Issues for Prioritizing Control Strategies', *Indian Journal of Occupational and Environmental Medicine*, 15(3): 93–96.

Kurian, N.J. and Sathymala, C. (2008). 'Health Sector in India: Issues and Challenges' in *India Social Development Report: Development and Displacement*, New Delhi: Oxford University Press

Larkin, M. (2011). *Social Aspects of Health, Illness and Healthcare*, New York: Open University Press.

Leslie, C. (1968). 'Professionalization of Ayurvedic and Unani Medicine', *Transactions of the New York Academy of Sciences, Series II*, 30(4): 559–572.

Levine, S. (1987). 'The Changing Terrains in Medical Sociology: Emergent Concerns with Quality of Life', *Journal of Health and Social Behaviour*, 28 (March): 1–6.

Lewis, O. (1958). *Village Life in Northern India*, New York: Random House.

Link, B.G. and Phelan, J. (1995). 'Social Conditions as Fundamental Causes of Disease', *Journal of Health and Social Behaviour*, 35 (extra issue): 80–94.

Lupton, D. (1996). *The Imperative of Health: Public Health and the Regulated Body*, London: Sage Publications.

——. (2003). *Medicine as Culture; Illness, Disease and the Body in Western Societies*, second edition, London: Sage Publications.

Madan, T.N. (1969). 'Who Chooses Modern Medicine and Why', *Economic and Political Weekly*, 4(37): 1475–1484.

——. (1972). 'Doctors in a North Indian City: Recruitment, Role Perception and Role Performance', in Saberwal, S. (ed.), *Beyond the Village: Sociological Explorations* (pp. 79–110), Shimla: Indian Institute of Advanced Study.

——. (1980). *Doctors and Society: Three Asian Case Studies (India, Malaysia and Sri Lanka)*, New Delhi: Vikas Publishing House.

Malvi, B.L. (1980). 'Venereal Diseases in Dungarpur District', *Tribe* (Special Number), 12(2–4): 36–48.

Mandal, A.K. (2009). 'Strategies and Policies Deteriorate Occupational Health Situation in India: A Review Based on Social Determinant Framework', *Indian Journal of Occupational and Environmental Medicine*, 13(3): 113–120.

Mane, P. and Maitra, S.A. (1992). *AIDS Prevention: The Socio-cultural Context in India*. Bombay: Tata Institute of Social Sciences.

Marmot, M. (2006). 'Social Causes of Social Inequalities in Health', in Anand, S., Peter, F. and Sen, A. (eds.), *Public Health, Ethics and Equity*, New Delhi: Oxford University Press.

Marriot, M. (1955). 'Western Medicine in a Village of Northern India', in Paul, B.D. (ed.), *Health, Culture and Community* (pp. 239–68), New York: Russel Sage Foundation.

Mathers, C., et al. (1999). *The Burden of Disease and Injury in Australia: Summary*, Canberra: Australian Institute of Health and Welfare.

Mathews, C.M.E and Benjamin, V. (1981). *Changing Health Beliefs and Practices in Rural Tamil Nadu*, New Delhi: Indian Social Institute.

Mathews, C.M.E. (1979). *Health and Culture in a South Indian Village*, New Delhi: Sterling.

Mathur, I. (1975). *Interrelations in an Organisation: A Study in Sociology of Medicine*. Jaipur: Aalekh Publishers.

McKenzie, J.F., Pinger, R.R. and Kotecki, J.E. (2002). *An Introduction to Community Health*, fourth edition, Massachusetts: Jones and Bartlett Publishers.

——. (2005). *An Introduction to Community Health*, London: Jones and Bartlett Publishers.

McNeill, P. (1990). *Health*, London: Routledge Publications.

Mechanic, D. (1978). *Medical Sociology*, New York: The Free Press.

Mehta, S.R. (1982). 'Sociology of Health and Medical Care: Research Needs and Challenges', in Nayar, P.K.B. (ed.), *Sociology of India* (pp. 301–328), New Delhi: B.R. Publishing Corp.

Miller, C., Waning, B., Bread, J. and Knapp, A. (2002). *Social Epidemiology, Chapter 2*, London: Jones and Bartlett Publishers.

Ministry of Health and Family Welfare, Government of India, official website.

Ministry of Health and Family Welfare, Government of India, The Journey So Far 2005–10, NRHM: Meeting People's Health Needs in Partnership with States, 2010.

Minocha (Ahluwalia), A. (1967). 'Sociology of Medicine in India: An Approach', *Economic and Political Weekly*, 2(22): 1007–1012.

Minocha (Ahluwalia), A. (1974). 'Sociology of Medicine', in M.N. Srinivas, M.S.A. Rao, and A.M. Shah (eds.), *A Survey of Research in Sociology and Social Anthropology*, Vol. II (pp. 401–430). Bombay: Popular Prakashan.

Minocha, A. (1980). 'Medical Pluralism and Health Services in India', *Social Science and Health*, 14B: 217–223.

——. (1991). 'Socio-economic Equity and Health: Examination of a Few Key Concepts', in Dak, T.M. (ed.), *Sociology of Health in India* (pp. 173–176), Jaipur: Rawat Publications.

——. (2010). 'The Socio-cultural Context of Informed Consent in Medical Practice', in Baviskar, B.S. and Patel, T. (eds.), *Understanding Indian Society: Past and Present* (pp. 257–279), New Delhi: Orient Blackswan.

Mishra, A. (ed.). (2010). *Health, Illness and Medicine: Ethnographic Readings*, New Delhi: Orient Blackswan.

Mishra, R.P. (2007). *Geography of Health*, Delhi: Concept Publications.

Mishra, V.K., Lahiri, S. and Luther, N.Y. (1999). 'Child Nutrition in India', National Family Health Survey Subject Reports, Number 14, June International Institute for Population Sciences Mumbai, India.

Mmom, P.C. and Mmom, C.F. (2011). 'Environmental Sanitation and Public Health Challenges in a Rapidly Growing City of the Third World: The Case of Domestic Waste and Diarrhoea Incidence in Greater Port Harcourt Metropolis, Nigeria', *Asian Journal of Medical Sciences*, 3 (3).

MoHFW. (2010). Annual Report to the People on Health, Government of India, Ministry of Health and Family welfare, September 2010.

Mukhopadhyay, I. (2008). 'Analyzing Health Inequalities: Social Capital and Its Infirmities', *Social Scientist*, 36(11–12): 69–93.

Müllegger, E., Langergraber, G. and Lechner, M. (2011). 'Sustainable Sanitation Practice, Planning Tools: Sustainable Sanitation Practice', *EcoSanClub*, Issue 7.

Murthy, M.S.R. (1993). *Sex Awareness among Rural Girls*, Delhi: B.R. Publishing Corp.

Nag, M. (1994). 'Sexual Behaviour and AIDS in India: State-of-the-Art', *The Indian Journal of Social Work*, LV(4): 617–632.

——. (1995). 'Sexual Behaviour in India with Risk of HIV/AIDS Transmission', *Health Transition Review*, 5: 293–305.

Nagla, B.K. and Nagla, M. (1991). 'Sociology of Health Policy in India', in Dak, T.M. (ed.), *Sociology of Health in India* (pp. 44–69), Jaipur: Rawat Publications.

Nagla, M. (1991). 'Patient and His Illness: A Sociological Analysis', in Dak, T.M. (ed.), *Sociology of Health in India* (pp. 123–141), Jaipur: Rawat Publications.

——. (1997). *Sociology of Medical Profession*, Jaipur: Rawat Publications.

National Family Health Survey (NFHS–3), 2005–06. (2007). India: International Institute for Population Sciences (IIPS) and Macro International. Vol. I. Mumbai: IIPS.

NCMEH. (2005). Report of the National Commission on Macroeconomics and Health, Ministry of Health and Family Welfare, Government of India, New Delhi, August.

Nettleton, S. (1995). *The Sociology of Health and Illness*, UK: Polity Press.

Norman, D., Kennedy, B., and Kawachi, I. (2006). 'Health and Inequality, or, Why Justice is Good for Our Health', in Anand, S., Peter, F., and Sen, A. (eds.), *Public Health, Ethics and Equity*, New Delhi: Oxford University Press.

OECD. (2010). *Health at a Glance: Asia/Pacific 2010*, OECD Publishing. Available online at: http://dx.doi.org/ 10.1787/9789264096202–en.

Oommen, T.K. (1978). *Doctors and Nurses: A Study in Occupational Role Structures*. Delhi: Macmillan.

Opler, E.M. (1963). 'The Cultural Definition of Illness in Village India', *Human Organisation*, 22(1): 32–35.

Pallikadavath S., Foss, M., Stones, R.W. (2004). 'Antenatal Care: Provision and Inequality in Rural North India', *Social Science and Medicine*, 59: 1147–1158.

Panikar, P.G.K. (1976). 'Health Care Delivery System in India: Alternative Approaches', *Economic and Political Weekly*, 11(22): 817–819.

Park, K. (2005). *Preventive and Social Medicine* 18th edition, Jabalpur: Banarsidas Bhanot.

——. (2009). *Preventive and Social Medicine* 20th edition, Jabalpur: Banarsidas Bhanot.

Parsons, T. (1972). 'Definitions of Health and Illness in the Light of American Values and Social Structure', in Jaco, E.G. (ed.), *Patients, Physicians, and Illness*, New York: McMillan Publications.

Pasrija, P., Sharma, M.L., and Sharma, A. (1991). 'Health Care Delivery System: A Sociological Analysis', in Dak, T.M. (ed.), *Sociology of Health in India* (pp. 142–161), Jaipur: Rawat Publications.

Patel, T. (2007). *Sex-selective Abortion in India*, Delhi: Sage Publications.

Pescosolido, B.A., Martin, J.K., McLeod, J.D. and Rogers, A. (2011). *Handbook of the Sociology of Health, Illness, and Healing: A Blueprint for the 21st Century*, New York: Springer.

Peter, F. (2006). 'Health Equity and Social Justice', in Anand, S., Peter, F., and Sen, A. (eds.), *Public Health, Ethics and Equity*, New Delhi: Oxford University Press.

Petersen, A. and Waddell, C. (1998). *Health Matters: A Sociology of Illness, Prevention and Care*, Sydney: Allen and Unwin.

Planning Commission. (2011). *Report of the Working Group on Disease Burden for the 12th Five-year plan: WGS 3 (1): Communicable Diseases*, No. 2 (6) 2010–H&FW, Government of India. Available online at: http://planningcommission.nic.in/aboutus/committee/wrkgrp12/health/WG_3_1communicable.pdf.

Porta, M. (2008). *A Dictionary of Epidemiology*, fifth edition, New York: Oxford, p. 68.

Prasad, B.G. (1963). 'Some Common Beliefs and Customs in Relation to Health and Diseases in Uttar Pradesh', *The Antiseptic*, 58: 225–238.

Qadeer, I. (1985). 'Health Service System in India: An Expression of Socio-Economic Inequalities' *Social Action*, 35.

——. (1991). 'Beyond Medicine: An Analysis of Health Status of Indian People', in Dak, T.M. (ed.), *Sociology of Health in India* (pp. 177–195), Jaipur: Rawat Publications.

——. (2001). 'Impact of Structural Adjustment Programme on Concepts in Public Health', in Qadeer, I., Sen, K. and Nayar, K.R. (eds.), *Public Health and the Poverty of Reforms: The South Asian Predicament* (pp. 117–156). New Delhi: Sage Publications.

Qadeer, I. and Nayar, K.R. (2005). 'Politics of Pedagogy in Public Health', *Social Scientist*, 33(1–2): 47–75.

Qadeer, I. and Priyadarshi, A.P. (2005). 'Nutrition Policy-shift and Logical Fallacies', *Economic and Political Weekly*, XL(5): 358–364.

Raj, H. (2007). *Fundamentals of Demography*, New Delhi: Surjeet Publications.

Rajora, P.D. (1990). *Community Culture and Health among the Bhils of Southern Rajasthan* (Unpublished Ph.D. Thesis), Udaipur: MLSU.

Rakesh, A. (1983). *Premarital Sexual Attitudes and Behaviour among Adolescent Girls*, Jaipur: Printwell.

Ramanamma, A. and Bambawale, U. (1978). 'Occupational Attitude of Physicians', *Sociological Bulletin*, 27(2): 190–207.

Ramani, K.V. and Dileep, Mavalankar. (n.d.). *Health System in India: Opportunities and Challenges for Improvement*, Ahmedabad: Indian Institute of Management.

Ramani, K.V., Mavalankar, D., Joshi, S., Malek, I., Puvar, T. and Kumar, H. (2010), 'Why Should 5,000 Children Die in India Every Day? Major Causes of Death and Managerial Challenges', *Vikalpa*, 35(2).

Rao, A., Nag, M., Mishra, K., et al. (1994). 'Sexual Behaviour Patterns of Truck Drivers and Their Helpers in Relation to Female Sex Workers'. *Indian Journal of Social Work*, 55(4): 603–615.

Rao, M. (2000). 'Family Planning Programme: Paradigm Shift in Strategy', *Economic and Political Weekly*, 35(49): 4317–4322.

Rao, T.V. (1977). *Doctors in Making,* Ahmedabad: Sahitya Mudranalay.

Raphael, D., Bryant, T., and Rioux, M. (ed.). (2006). *Staying Alive: Critical Perspectives on Health, Illness, and Health Care,* Toronto, Ontario: Canadian Scholars' Press Inc.

Rastogi, R. (1981). *Social Status and Use of Medical System* (Unpublished Ph.D. Thesis), Varanasi: BHU.

Rizvi, S.N.H. (1986). 'Health Practices of the Jaunsaris: A Socio-cultural Analysis', in Chaudhuri, B. (ed.), *Tribal Health: Socio-cultural Dimensions* (pp. 85–98), New Delhi: Inter-India Publication.

Robeyns, I. (2006). 'Sen's Capability Approach and Gender Inequality: Selecting Relevant Capabilities', in Agarwal, B., Humphires, J. and Robeyns, I. (eds.), *Capability, Freedom and Equality: Amartya Sen's Work from a Gender Perspective*, New Delhi: Oxford University Press.

Roy, R.U., Basu, U., Mukhapadhya, S., et al. (1999). 'Mother and Child Care among Some Kharia Community in Similipal Area, Orissa', in Behera, D.K. and Pfeffer, G. (eds.), *Contemporary Society: Tribal Studies* (pp. 293–309), New Delhi: Concept Publishing Company.

Rural Sanitation and Health Booklet No. 416, Health and Medicine: HMS—2.

Saha, U.C. and Saha, K.B. (2010). 'A Trend in Women's Health in India: What Has Been Achieved and What Can Be Done', *Rural and Remote Health*. Available online at: http://www.rrh.org.au.

Savara, M. and Sridhar, C.R. (1994). 'Sexual Behaviour amongst Different Occupational Groups in Maharashtra, India and the Implications for AIDS Education', *Indian Journal of Social Work,* 55(4): 617–632.

Scambler, G. (ed.). (1987). *Sociological Theory and Medical Sociology*, London: Tavistock Publications.

Schoenbach, V.J. and Rosamond, W.D. (2000). *Understanding the Fundamentals of Epidemiology: An Evolving Text*, Department of Epidemiology, School of public Health, University of North Carolina.

Scott, J. (2006). *Sociology: The Key Concepts*, London/New York: Routledge, Taylor and Francis Group

Segel, J.E. (2006). *Cost-of-Illness Studies: A Primer*, RTI International, RTI-UNC Center of Excellence in Health Promotion Economics.

Sen, A. (2006a). 'Health Achievement and Equity: External and Internal Perspectives,' in Anand, S., Peter, F. and Sen, A. (eds.), *Public Health, Ethics and Equity*, New Delhi: Oxford University Press.

——. (2006b). 'Development as Capability Expansion', in Agarwal, B., Humphires, J. and Robeyns, I. (eds.), *Capability, Freedom and Equality: Amartya Sen's Work from a Gender Perspective*, New Delhi: Oxford University Press.

——. (2006c). 'Why Health Equity?', in Anand, S., Peter, F. and Sen, A. (eds.), *Public Health, Ethics and Equity*, New Delhi: Oxford University Press.

Sharadamma, S. and Parvathamma, C. (1968). 'Some Aspects of Socio-economic and Political Background of Medical Students in Mysore', *Arts Journal of the Mysore University*, 24: 49–56.

Sharma, M. (1991). 'Women and Health: Problems and Issues', in Dak, T.M. (ed.), *Sociology of Health in India* (pp. 196–216), Jaipur: Rawat Publications.

Sheaff, M. (2005). *Sociology and Health Care: An Introduction for Nurses, Midwives and Allied Health Professionals*, New York: Open University Press.

Singh, B. (1995). 'An Overview of Tribal Health', in Singh, B. and Mohanty, N. (eds.), *Tribal Health in India* (pp. 17–32), New Delhi: Inter-India Publication.

Singh, Y. (2004). *Ideology and Theory in Indian Sociology*, Jaipur: Rawat Publications.

Sinha, S. (1958). 'Training of a Bhumij Medicine-Man', *Man in India*, 38(2): 111–128.

Srivastava, A.L. (1976). *Doctor-Patient Relationship in Hospital Situation* (Unpublished Ph.D. Thesis), Varanasi: BHU.

Stacey, M. and Homans, H. (1978). 'The Sociology of Health and Illness: Its Present State, Future Prospect and Potential for Health Research', *Sociology*, 12(2): 281–307.

Stephenson, J., Bauman, A., Armstrong, T., et al. (2000). *The Costs of Illness Attributable to Physical Inactivity in Australia: A Preliminary Study*, Population Health Division Publications, p. 2.

Stolley, K.S. (2005). *The Basics of Sociology*, USA: Greenwood Publishing Group.

Straus, R. (1957). 'The Nature and Status of Medical Sociology', *American Sociological Review,* 22: 200–204.

Sujatha, V. (2002). 'Food: The Immanent Cause from Outside. Medical Lore on Food and Health in Village Tamil Nadu', *Sociological Bulletin,* 51(1): 80–100.

——. (2003). *Health by the People: Sociology of Medical Lore,* Jaipur: Rawat Publications.

——. (2007). 'Pluralism in Indian Medicine: Medical Lore as a Genre of Medical Knowledge', *Contributions to Indian Sociology,* 41(2): 169–202.

Talukia, H.S., Taylor, E.E., et al. (1967). *The Health Centre Doctor in India,* Baltimore: The John Hopkins Press.

Thomas, R.K. (2002). *Society and Health: Sociology for Health Professionals,* New York: Kluwer Academic Publishers.

Tillman, C. (ed.). (2007). *Principles of Occupational Health and Hygiene: An Introduction.* Australia: Allen & Unwin Publication.

Timmappaya, A., et al. (1971). *Patient Satisfaction and Ward Social System* (NIHAE research monograph), New Delhi: National Institute of Health Administration and Education.

Tischler, H.L. (2011). *Introduction to Sociology,* tenth edition, USA: Wadsworth, Cengage Learning.

Tiwari, T.R., et al. (1971). *An Exploratory Study of Integrated Health Services in India* (NIHAE research monograph), New Delhi: National Institute of Health Administration and Education.

Turner, B. (2006). *The Cambridge Dictionary of Sociology,* Cambridge: Cambridge University Press.

Venkataratnam, R. (1979). *Medical Sociology in an Indian Setting,* Madras: Macmillan.

Vyas, N.N. (1980). 'Cultural Background of Venereal Disease', in N.N. Vyas and R.S. Mann (eds.), *Disease, Culture Contact and Tribals,* Udaipur: The Tribal Research and Training Institute.

Wainwright, D. (2008). *A Sociology of Health,* London, New Delhi: Sage Publications.

Wall, A. and Owen, B. (2005). *Health Policy,* second edition, London/New York: Routledge Publications.

Weitz, R. (2012). *The Sociology of Health, Illness, and Healthcare: A Critical Approach,* sixth edition, Boston: Wadsworth Cengage Learning.

White, K. (2002). *An Introduction to the Sociology of Health and Illness,* London: Sage Publications.

——. (2006). *SAGE Dictionary of Health and Society,* New Delhi: Sage Publications.

——. (2009). *An Introduction to the Sociology of Health and Illness*, second edition, London: Sage Publications.

WHO. (1952). *Report of Expert Committee on Public Health Administration.*

WHO. (2010). *The world health report: health systems financing: The path to universal coverage*. Available online at: www.who.int/entity/whr/2010/overview.pdf (accessed 5 July 2012).

Wilkinson, R. and Mormot, M. (2003). *Social Determinants of Health: The Solid Facts*, second edition, International Centre for Health and society. WHO available at: http://www.euro.who.int/__data/assets/pdf_file/0005/98438/e81384.pdf

World Health Organization. (2003). 'Right to Water', Health and Human Rights Publication Series; no. 3, World Health Organization.

World Health Organization. (2011). *Non-communicable diseases country profiles 2011*. Available online at: http://whqlibdoc. who.int/publications/2011/9789241502283_eng.pdf.

Yuill, C. (2005). 'Marx: Capitalism, Alienation and Health, *Social Theory and Health*, 3, 126–143, Palgrave Macmillan Ltd.

Websites

en.wikipedia.org/wiki/Sanitation

http://davidscottsociology.tripod.com

http://dx.doi.org/10.1787/9789264096202–en

http://en.wikipedia.org/wiki/Medical_sociology

http://en.wikipedia.org/wiki/Sociology_of_health

http://medical-dictionary.thefreedictionary.com/illness+experience

http://medicina.kmu.lt/0702/0702–04e.pdf

http://webtools.delmarlearning.com/sample_chapters/marotz_ch01.pdf

http://www.healthizen.com/blog/index.php/general/environmental-sanitation/

http://www.medicalnewstoday.com/articles/150999.php

http://www.rsby.gov.in/about_rsby.html

http://www.who.int/social_determinants/tools/multimedia/alma_ata/en/index.html

whqlibdoc.who.int/publications/a38153_(ch21).pdf.

www.bmj.com/content/324/7342/859.full

www.jeywin.com

www.newagepublishers.com/samplechapter/000315.pdf

www.palgrave.com/bilton/pdfs/0333_945719_14_cha13.pdf

Index